Nursing Case Studies in Caring

Charlotte D. Barry, PhD, RN, NCSN, FAAN, is a professor at the Christine E. Lynn College of Nursing, Florida Atlantic University, in Boca Raton, Florida. Nationally certified in school nursing, Dr. Barry's outstanding and sustained contribution to nursing has been the outcome of her expertise in community nursing practice, education, and research. She has been on the leading edge of developing school-based health centers dedicated to overcoming barriers in the delivery of quality care to children and families.

As co-director of the Center for School and Community Well-Being, she secured over $7 million in grants and contracts to fund nurse-managed school-based wellness centers and school nurse education programs in the southeastern United States. The nurse-managed centers in schools often provide the only ongoing access to health care for many children and families. The outcomes of improved health, return-to-class rate, and attendance served as the impetus for a substantial and sustained policy change, resulting in a school nurse present at every public school in one of the largest school districts in the United States, serving over 176,000 students.

Dr. Barry has transformed nursing practice through curricula change, community immersion, and policy development. Her publications and presentations at national and international conferences have fostered understanding of the value of caring for the most vulnerable and have impacted the professional practice of school nursing, now recognized as an expert practice and venue for access to affordable and ongoing health care for children and families in the United States, Africa, and Haiti.

Shirley C. Gordon, PhD, RN, NCSN, is a professor and assistant dean of graduate practice programs at the Christine E. Lynn College of Nursing at Florida Atlantic University. She is actively involved in teaching research, theory, ethics, and community nursing to both undergraduate and graduate students. Her research areas of interest include caring for persons experiencing chronic, stigmatized conditions; the development of caring theories to guide nursing practice; and teaching from nursing situations.

Dr. Gordon's sustained contribution to nursing has been as an international leader in caring for children and families with persistent head lice. She is the first researcher to study the impact of persistent head lice on families and named the phenomenon *persistent head lice*, which she defined as distinct from resistant head lice. Her groundbreaking research and midrange theory development have transformed how persons with head lice are perceived and have influenced policy development, nursing curricula, and programs of research. Nationally certified in school nursing, Dr. Gordon serves as the founder and director of the Head Lice Treatment and Prevention Project and is actively involved in the direct care of children and families experiencing head lice.

Dr. Gordon has multiple publications in national and international nursing journals and has received national funding to support her research and service efforts in the areas of persistent head lice, disability, genital herpes, Bell's palsy, delegation, and school nursing. Dr. Gordon was recognized in 2010 as one of the Great 100 Nurses in the State of Florida in the area of research.

Beth M. King, PhD, RN, PMHCNS-BC, is an assistant professor at the Christine E. Lynn College of Nursing. Nationally certified as a clinical nurse specialist in adult psychiatric and mental health, her area of focus is community practice and mental health. Her research areas of interest are caring outcomes in nursing education and the burden of depression in vulnerable and often marginalized populations.

Certified as a HeartMath® trainer, Dr. King has been working with undergraduate nursing students to enhance resilience skills needed for day-to-day nursing practice. She has been recognized for countless hours of voluntary service to boards and communities in the United States and Haiti, including participating in the development of a school-based health center in Haiti. This center is providing access to health care for children and families in a rural, underserved community.

Dr. King has received funding to support her research in the areas of nursing education outcomes related to caring and school nursing. Her presentations and publications on the use of nursing situations as a teaching method have inspired the transformation of nursing education focused on the study of caring in contextualized stories from practice.

Nursing Case Studies in Caring

Across the Practice Spectrum

Charlotte D. Barry, PhD, RN, NCSN, FAAN
Shirley C. Gordon, PhD, RN, NCSN
Beth M. King, PhD, RN, PMHCNS-BC

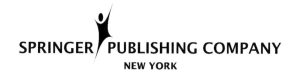
SPRINGER PUBLISHING COMPANY
NEW YORK

Springer Publishing Company, LLC
11 West 42nd Street
New York, NY 10036
www.springerpub.com

Acquisitions Editor: Joseph Morita
Production Editor: Kris Parrish
Composition: Exeter Premedia Services Private Ltd.

ISBN: 978-0-8261-7178-8
e-book ISBN: 978-0-8261-7179-5

16 17 18 / 5 4 3 2

The author and the publisher of this Work have made every effort to use sources believed to be reliable to provide information that is accurate and compatible with the standards generally accepted at the time of publication. Because medical science is continually advancing, our knowledge base continues to expand. Therefore, as new information becomes available, changes in procedures become necessary. We recommend that the reader always consult current research and specific institutional policies before performing any clinical procedure. The author and publisher shall not be liable for any special, consequential, or exemplary damages resulting, in whole or in part, from the readers' use of, or reliance on, the information contained in this book. The publisher has no responsibility for the persistence or accuracy of URLs for external or third-party Internet websites referred to in this publication and does not guarantee that any content on such websites is, or will remain, accurate or appropriate.

Library of Congress Cataloging-in-Publication Data

Nursing case studies in caring : across the practice spectrum / [edited by] Charlotte D. Barry, Shirley C. Gordon, Beth M. King.
    p. ; cm.
    Includes bibliographical references.
    ISBN 978-0-8261-7178-8—ISBN 978-0-8261-7179-5 (eISBN)
    I. Barry, Charlotte D., editor.   II. Gordon, Shirley C., 1953- , editor.   III. King, Beth M., editor.
    [DNLM: 1. Nursing Care—psychology—Case Reports.   2. Empathy—Case Reports.   3. Nurse-Patient Relations—Case Reports. WY 87]
    RT41
    610.73—dc23

                                                                              2015002722

Printed in the United States of America by Gasch Printing.

Contents

Contributors

Alana Andrews, BSN, RN Graduate Student, Florida Atlantic University, Christine E. Lynn College of Nursing, Boca Raton, Florida

Fortunate Atwine, MNsc, RN, ICN Lecturer, Mbarara University of Science and Technology, Mbarara, Uganda

Christie Bailey, MS, RN, AHN-BC PhD Student, Florida Atlantic University, Christine E. Lynn College of Nursing, Boca Raton, Florida

Anne Boykin, PhD, RN Director, Anne Boykin Institute for the Advancement of Caring in Nursing, Boca Raton, Florida

Shelina Davis, ARNP, GNP-BC Vice President of Operations, Florida East Coast Health, LLC, Cocoa, Florida

Margarita Dorsey, BSN, RN, CCRN DNP Student, Florida Atlantic University, Christine E. Lynn College of Nursing, Boca Raton, Florida

Valarie Grumme, MSN, RN, CCRN Clinical Manager MICU/CCU, Memorial Regional Hospital, Hollywood, Florida; PhD student, Florida Atlantic University, Christine E. Lynn College of Nursing, Boca Raton, Florida

Debra Hain, PhD, ARNP, ANP-BC, GNP-BC, FAANP Associate Professor, Florida Atlantic University, Christine E. Lynn College of Nursing, Boca Raton, Florida; Nurse Practitioner, Cleveland Clinic Florida, Department of Nephrology, Weston, Florida

Molly Johnson, EdS, ASN, RN Graduate Student, Florida Atlantic University, Christine E. Lynn College of Nursing, Boca Raton, Florida

Patricia Blanchette Kronk, MSN, ARNP, GNP-BC Geriatric Nurse Practitioner, The Villages, Florida

Bernadette Lange, PhD, RN, AHN-BC Associate Professor, Florida Atlantic University, Christine E. Lynn College of Nursing, Boca Raton, Florida

Karmel McCarthy-Riches, MAOM, BSN, RN Graduate Student, Florida Atlantic University, Christine E. Lynn College of Nursing, Boca Raton, Florida

Alina Miracle, DNP, ARNP, FNP-C DNP Student, Florida Atlantic University, Christine E. Lynn College of Nursing, Boca Raton, Florida

Michelle Palokas, DNP, RN-CPN Inpatient Clinical Director, Children's of Mississippi, Jackson, Mississippi

Dana Reynolds, BSN, RN Graduate Student, Florida Atlantic University, Christine E. Lynn College of Nursing, Boca Raton, Florida

Rosemary Schiel, BSN, RN, CCM, CPHM Director of Case Management, West Boca Medical Center, West Boca, Florida

Savina O. Schoenhofer, PhD, RN Retired Nurse Educator; Member, Board of Anne Boykin Institute for the Advancement of Caring in Nursing, Boca Raton, Florida

Michael Shaw, BSN, RN Mississippi State Hospital, Whitfield, Mississippi; Graduate Student, University of Mississippi Medical Center, Jackson, Mississippi

Arthur L. Tailleur, MDiv, BSN, RN HCA Gulf Coast Division IT&S, Houston, Texas

Mary Ellen Wright, PhD, APRN, CPNP Nurse Researcher, Women's and Children's Health, Mission Health, Asheville, North Carolina

Foreword

Nursing education is in the process of radical transformation. We can no longer call ourselves a professional discipline without engaging students in learning the content of that discipline. We can no longer sustain the great divide between didactic and practice (clinical) learning and expect graduates to see the value of theory-guided practice. We can no longer spew out facts and formulae for care to be ingested by our students and regurgitated back to us and then question why graduates cannot think critically. In this new era of nursing education, we educators must create learning opportunities where students integrate nursing science and art. Students need to learn through immersion in both real and virtual situations of care, where they can apply the generalities of the theoretical to the particularities of the "real" situation. Simulation is one method of approaching this integration. Another approach is to engage students in the study of nursing through stories of real or imagined encounters with clients (individuals, families, groups, and communities).

The Carnegie Foundation for the Advancement of Teaching's report, *Educating Nurses: A Call for Radical Transformation* (Benner, Sutphen, Leonard, & Day, 2010), recommends four essential shifts for more effective integration of nursing science and caring practices: "(a) Shift from a focus on covering decontextualized knowledge to an emphasis on teaching for a sense of salience, situation cognition and action in particular situations; (b) Shift from a sharp separation of clinical and classroom teaching to integration of classroom and clinical teaching; (c) Shift from an emphasis on critical thinking to an emphasis on clinical reasoning and multiple ways of thinking that include critical thinking; (d) Shift from an emphasis on socialization and role-taking to an emphasis on formation" (p. 89). This groundbreaking book offers an approach to teaching/learning that embodies these four transformative shifts. The book contains nursing situations featuring diverse populations, health concerns, and settings. By engaging with these situations, students learn the salient knowledge of the discipline of nursing by actively reasoning within the particularities of these situations. These nursing situations are stories of practice that can be used in the classroom to bridge the gap between theory and practice. The authors encourage the use of a framework for approaching the study of these nursing situations through multiple ways of knowing, and these include both critical and creative thinking. Through engagement with the nursing situations, students are called to imagine themselves being in the situation, reflecting on their thoughts, feelings, and perceptions. In this process, students come to a deeper understanding of themselves and the fullness of nursing grounded in caring.

The authors of this book, Drs. Charlotte Barry, Shirley Gordon, and Beth King, are faculty of Florida Atlantic University's Christine E. Lynn College of Nursing. I am privileged to be the dean of this unique college, whose mission has focused on advancing the science, art, and study of caring within the discipline of nursing since the early 1980s. In 1994, Dr. Anne Boykin, former dean of the college, edited the book *Living a Caring-Based Program* (Boykin, 1994), in which the faculty at that time explicated a caring-based approach to teaching/learning nursing; it included using the nursing situation as the foundation for the study of nursing. Although faculty at the college have been committed to teaching using nursing situations for some time, the actual "how to" has been challenging. With this book, we have the structure and raw material that is needed to teach successfully from nursing situations throughout the curriculum. I am so grateful to and proud of these creative scholars for their exquisite work on this book.

The volume is organized to guide the reader through the process of understanding and applying this approach to teaching/learning. The authors' perspective is that caring is the central domain of nursing; therefore, their approach to the study of the nursing situations is through the explicit lens of caring. Chapter 1 orients the reader to the concept of a nursing situation as a vehicle for the study of the discipline of nursing. Chapter 2 provides the philosophical and theoretical foundation in caring, knowing, and the use of stories for the study of nursing situations. Chapter 3 offers the reader a clear and practical framework for studying nursing situations using ways of knowing and calls for nursing. In Chapter 4, the authors provide a framework for integrating nursing theories (nursing's disciplinary knowledge) into the context of the study of nursing situations. The following chapters (5 through 20) include the actual nursing situations, shared by a variety of contributors, as well as focused questions and study processes. This elegant guide is useful to any educators wanting to use a contextualized approach to teach nursing in their courses.

This seminal work provides what is needed for educators to take the next step in revolutionizing nursing education. Educators throughout the world in academic and practice settings, eager to teach and study caring and healing, will find this book essential. The approach of studying nursing through these nursing situations can accommodate diverse theoretical perspectives and levels of nursing education, from beginning students to staff development to graduate students. This book will become a critical resource for both novice and seasoned teachers. I have been wishing, hoping, and waiting for this book for some time. Now that it is here, I offer my most sincere "thank you" to Drs. Barry, Gordon, and King for this transformative gift to those committed to teaching and studying nursing.

Marlaine C. Smith, PhD, RN, AHN-BC, FAAN
Dean and Helen K. Persson Eminent Scholar
Florida Atlantic University
Christine E. Lynn College of Nursing
Boca Raton, Florida

REFERENCES

Benner, P., Sutphen, M., Leonard, V., & Day, L. (2010). *Educating nurses: A call for radical transformation.* San Francisco, CA: Jossey-Bass.

Boykin, A. (1994). *Living a caring-based program.* New York, NY: National League for Nursing.

Preface

This book provides a transformative approach to the study of nursing through nursing case studies in caring, described in this book as nursing situations. Grounded in the foundational belief that caring is the central domain of nursing, this book provides an innovative and exciting approach to the study of nursing from within the context of nursing situations. Nursing situations are defined as the shared lived experience in which the caring between the nurse and the one nursed nurtures wholeness and well-being.

The title of the book, *Nursing Case Studies in Caring: Across the Practice Spectrum*, has drawn us into deep reflection on the meaning of the concepts of case study, nursing case study in caring, and nursing situation. A traditional understanding of *case studies* as a teaching modality is drawn from the discipline of medicine in which the focus historically has been on disease, medical management, and cure. The term *nursing case studies in caring* is intended to denote a more holistic approach using multiple ways of knowing and caring science to inform the study of nursing. To avoid conceptual confusion, we prefer the simple language of the construct *nursing situation* to capture the disciplinary focus, to illuminate caring relationships, and to distinguish from the multidisciplinary use of the term *case study*. We will use the term throughout the text.

The Barry, Gordon & King Teaching/Learning Nursing Framework reflects the philosophy of Florida Atlantic University's Christine E. Lynne College of Nursing (2012) and was developed as a useful guide to uncover the knowledge and beauty of nursing embedded in nursing situations. However, the framework can be adapted to any philosophical or theoretical framework currently used in education or practice. Using multiple ways of knowing and understanding, the framework provides direct and reflective questions to assist in uncovering the content, structure, and meaning of the nursing situation for the nurse, the one nursed, nursing, and for others. This book is a core resource for nurse educators and students at all levels who seek to study the art and science of nursing grounded in caring. Additionally, the book is a resource for in-service educators in health care systems that specifically address caring as an essential value for practice.

We organized the chapters into two major parts. In Part I, "Foundational Concepts" (Chapters 1 through 5), we provide an introduction to the concept of nursing situations; an overview of the philosophical and theoretical perspectives grounding the framework development; an explanation of the Barry, Gordon & King Teaching/Learning Nursing Framework; a conceptual translation and application of the framework to selected grand and midrange theoretical perspectives; and an in-depth exemplar of teaching the discipline of nursing through the use of a nursing situation at the graduate level.

In Part II, "Nursing Situation Exemplars" (Chapters 6 through 20), we present examples of nursing situations across a variety of populations, health concerns, and practice settings that can be woven into a range of courses. The exemplars were selected from nursing situations gathered from nursing faculty and students over many years of teaching/learning nursing. Focused and reflective questions, designed to guide mutual student and faculty engagement and co-creation of nursing responses, are not intended to be exhaustive. We encourage the development of additional questions to guide understanding of caring between the nurse and one nursed. Suggested learning activities including journaling exercises, movie reviews, and aesthetic re-presentations are presented.

This book answers the clarion call for a framework from which nursing can be studied with contextualized stories from day-to-day practice. Teaching/learning from this perspective brings the lived experience of nursing into the "classroom" as students and faculty explore the impact of caring on health concerns experienced by individuals, families, and groups. We invite your responses to the usefulness of this framework for teaching/learning nursing from nursing situations.

Charlotte D. Barry
Shirley C. Gordon
Beth M. King

REFERENCE

Florida Atlantic University, Christine E. Lynn College of Nursing. (2012). *Philosophy*. Retrieved from http://nursing.fau.edu/index.php?main=1&nav=635

Acknowledgments

We are grateful to our role models and mentors, Drs. Anne Boykin, Savina Schoenhofer, and Marilyn Parker, who fueled our love of nursing with ideas and language, all the while inspiring us to reach higher and delve deeper into understanding the fullness of nursing, the liveliness of caring.

We are indebted to our many colleagues, faculty, and students who not only inspired the idea of the book but motivated and supported us in its design and creation.

PART I

Foundational Concepts

CHAPTER 1

Introduction to Nursing Case Studies in Caring as Nursing Situations

Grounded in the foundational belief that caring is the central domain of nursing, this book provides a distinctive transformative approach to the study of nursing through nursing case studies in caring, described as nursing situations. The authors intentionally use the simple language of the construct *nursing situation* in place of *nursing case studies in caring* to capture the disciplinary focus, illuminate caring relationships, and distinguish from the multidisciplinary use of the term *case study*. Nursing situations are stories from day-to-day practice defined as the shared lived experience in which caring between the nurse and the one nursed nurtures wholeness and well-being. Nursing situations reach beyond the medical story to incorporate multiple ways of knowing and understanding in caring for individuals, families, or groups. The nursing situations presented in this book illustrate a practical, dynamic approach to the study of nursing concepts at the undergraduate as well as the graduate level. Although nursing knowledge embedded in a nursing situation is contextual, the application of that knowledge to other nursing situations that are both similar and divergent is spectacularly unlimited. Nursing situations draw readers in—turning the focus away from the disease, desk, chart, doorway, or machine—with an urgency to touch, feel, participate with, and experience what it is like to be together at this moment, at this time, in this complex particularity (King, Barry, & Gordon, 2014). This is the foundation for understanding self and others as living caring in nursing situations and as the seedling to co-create nursing responses that nurture wholeness and well-being of persons and environment in caring (Florida Atlantic University, Christine

E. Lynn College of Nursing [FAU, CON], 2012). Individuals are unique and irreducible, interconnected with others and the environment in caring relationships. The nature of being human is to be caring. Humans choose values that give meaning to living and enhance well-being. Well-being is creating and living the meaning of life. From this lens, the individual defines what wholeness means to him or her, what is necessary for well-being, and what matters most at that time for the one nursed.

BACKGROUND

National groups and scholars (American Association of Colleges of Nursing [AACN], 2010; Benner, Sulphen, Leonard, & Day, 2010; The Carnegie Foundation, 2010; Chinn, 2014; Hills & Watson, 2011; Institute of Medicine, 2011; Kagen, Smith, Cowling, & Chinn, 2009; Sullivan, 2008; Watson, 2010) have called for transformation in the way nurses are educated; these include innovative educational approaches that help illuminate and unify the complex, divergent dimensions that must be studied in order to practice nursing thoughtfully and competently. In response to these calls, this book presents a framework to support the study of nursing situations, described as the "co-created lived experiences in which the caring between nurses and persons enhances well-being" (FAU, CON, 2012). The study of nursing situations allows the reader to uncover the knowledge, skills, and practices most relevant to the real-life, day-to-day practice of nursing. National reports, including the Phase I project overview from Quality Safety Education in Nursing (2005), Core Competencies for Nurse Educators (National League for Nursing [NLN], 2005), Core Competencies of Nurse Practitioners (National Organization of Nurses Practitioner Faculty [NONPF], 2011), *The Essentials of Baccalaureate Education for Professional Nursing Practice* (AACN, 2010), The Joint Commission's National Patient Safety Goals (2014), and Healthy People 2020 (U.S. Department of Health and Human Services, 2014), were analyzed to identify essential concepts related to nursing education for practice. As a result, the following concepts were identified and utilized for selection and inclusion of the nursing situations: (a) caring, (b) leadership, (c) patient safety, (d) evidence-based practice, (e) research/inquiry, (f) communication, (g) interprofessional collaboration, (h) health policy, (i) advocacy, (j) social justice, (k) health care disparities, and (l) professional values/ethics.

PEDAGOGICAL APPROACH

The pedagogical approach of this book to teaching/learning nursing is from a disciplinary perspective that caring is the central domain of nursing knowledge (Boykin & Schoenhofer, 2001; Leininger & McFarland, 2010; Newman,

Sime, & Corcoran-Perry, 1991; Smith, 2013; Swanson, 1991; Watson, 1979) and the belief that the knowledge of nursing is embedded in contextualized stories of practice nursing situations (Boykin & Schoenhofer, 2001; Paterson & Zderad, 1988; Touhy & Boykin, 2008). Nursing situations are examined using theoretical and philosophical perspectives of caring and various ways of exploring the meaning and practices of nursing by weaving together clinical and classroom experiences to assist the student in making the connection between theory, research, and practice.

The poem, "I Am Nurse" (see Box 1.1; Barry, 1990), as an aesthetic re-presentation of a nursing situation, illuminates the connection between theory, research, and practice. Aesthetic re-presentations, described in depth in Chapter 3, enable the student to use artistic expression to display the essence of caring from a nursing situation in a creative way. This poem is a stylized series of vignettes from the day-to-day practice of a home health nurse, and communicates the value of caring in nursing. This poem has been shared with students and colleagues around the globe and has elicited a common understanding of what is nursing and what it means to be a nurse.

Chapter 3 describes an innovative framework for teaching/learning nursing from nursing situations.

MULTIPLE APPROACHES TO TEACHING/LEARNING FROM NURSING SITUATIONS

The main theme of this book is that nursing situations constitute an ideal text–context configuration of details that focus the study of nursing science on the core value of nursing—which is caring—and integrates a range of relevant characteristics around that core. The following exemplars illustrate how nursing situations offer a "practical organic" approach to the study of nursing at the undergraduate as well as the graduate level. The exemplars are part of a data set gathered during a study of the usefulness of using nursing situations to teach nursing (King, Barry, & Gordon, 2014). A common thread of the experience of teaching using nursing situations was how nursing situations were woven into a range of courses revealing a tapestry of unique creativity.

One participant described nursing situations as the "bedrock of nursing education, practice, and research." She shared her use of students' nursing situations across a curriculum, but focused on a particular undergraduate course. In an early course, traditional students studied general nursing situations with "healthy" individuals of all ages. A corequisite practice course immersed the students in learning how to come to know and care for individuals in community-based settings such as preschools; elementary, middle, and high schools; older adult day care; and other congregate living facilities. Students wrote in their journals weekly, recording their reflections

BOX 1.1   Aesthetic Re-presentation: The Poem, "I Am Nurse"

By Charlotte D. Barry

I am nurse, my name is not remembered
But my caring practice names me nurse and defines nursing for my patients
I am nurse and I transcend the moment
With Bob and Mark
isolated from the world
and from each other by the cold iron bars of the hospital bed
I say— "Mark—get in bed with your partner and do it now
I know you understand the urgency
You know Bob's process of transcending this life
Get in bed and warm him and warm yourself."

I am nurse and I transcend the moment
With Meghan
Meghan is suffering with AIDS, a beautiful young woman
Reminds me of my daughter with her crisp good looks and hope for the future
I go through the process of admission to the home health agency and I ask this lovely
young married 32-year-old woman
"Do you have any problems with your heart?"
And she thinks for a moment and looks at me and says
"Only that my heart is broken."
And my heart breaks and we transcend the moment through my tears.

My name is nurse and I transcend the moment with Edith
Suffering with cancer of the liver, struggling with
The restraints of limited resources,
Unable to pay the rent since she's been sick,
Unable to get her TV repaired—her only diversion from her reality.
I transcend the moment by securing resources from the church, fellow nurses and
a woman suffering with cancer who understands
what it's like to have your back up against the wall
And Edith's last days are spent with a few dollars, sufficient food, a rent subsidy
and cable TV.

My name is nurse and I transcend the moment with Ann
Suffering with uterine cancer, isolation and fear—
She longs for the peace, hope and safety she felt in Brandenberg—
wishing she were there
I ask if she would like me to take her on a trip to a safe place, a place where she
could feel hope and healing and she agrees.
Through guided imagery we embark on a journey together toward the light of healing
and we're both transformed forever.

I am nurse
I live in my relations and
I grow and change by my relationships
And so does nursing but my name remains nurse.

on coming to know themselves and the one nursed as living caring in nursing situations. Works by Roach (1992) and Mayeroff (1971) were used to identify caring concepts, and Carper's "Fundamental Patterns of Knowing" (1978) linked knowledge needed to nurse an individual/group or family. The following is adapted from a student's journal:

> *Journal entry*: We were visiting a woman in a continuing care retirement community and having a conversation about her life. The woman shared that her eyesight was deteriorating and she could no longer write notes. We asked, "How can we be helpful to you?" and she asked us to help her write some long overdue notes. We agreed and my colleague went to find stationery and pen while I sat with the woman. I looked closely at the woman's eyeglasses and asked if it would be alright if I washed them; she said yes. I went to the sink, washed the eyeglasses and removed layers of what was later identified as hair spray film from the lenses. I returned the glasses to the woman, who put them on and was amazed and overjoyed that she could see again. We were also amazed and overjoyed that through our intention to care for her we could make such a difference with our simple nursing interaction. Back in the classroom we shared an aesthetic re-presentation of this nursing situation. We built a huge pair of wooden eyeglasses and decorated it with the words that exemplified caring in our nursing situation: *Knowing*, taking the time to sit and talk to this woman; *Compassion*, feeling her sadness at not being able to write to her family and friends anymore; and the *Courage* to ask if we could wash her glasses.

Another faculty described a different approach to teaching using nursing situations. In an undergraduate pharmacology course, this faculty flips the classroom. Lecture notes and reading assignments are uploaded on a website platform and students are expected to come prepared to apply principles of pharmacology to nursing situations. The faculty provides nursing situations from a broad practice perspective. The core caring ingredient is focused on caring for the one nursed by competence in not only knowing drugs, dosages, interactions, allergic reactions, and side effects, but also in understanding the context of the person's life. Issues such as literacy, health literacy, poverty, affordability, vision, refrigeration, availability of help, accessibility to a pharmacy, and manual dexterity stretches the students toward compassion and advocacy for access parity and health equity.

Similarly, the complexity of an undergraduate adult health nursing course is taught by faculty members who weave nursing situations into lectures. The students are challenged to reflect and integrate ways of caring and knowing with questions such as, "What would you do, if you were the nurse in the following nursing situation?"

Daisey was dying in the cardiac care unit. Her preacher wanted to visit and bring along other church members outside posted visiting hours. The nurse let them in a secret back door to the unit. The door to Daisey's room was closed to give them privacy and their singing gospel music was loud and soothing.

On reflection the nurse said, "If Daisey doesn't make it out of here we need to make sure her last hours are spent nurturing her wholeness and well-being."

Reflecting on another nursing situation, the students are challenged to think beyond asking the usual assessment questions of "How do you feel?" or "Did you have a good night?" or "How is your breathing today?" Alice, a concert pianist, was very ill. The nurse asked, "What matters most to you today?" Alice responded, "Playing the piano, but I don't think I ever will again." Hearing this distinct call for nursing, the nurse enlisted the help of colleagues, a piano was rolled from the lobby to the hall outside the patient's room, and Alice sat down and played. The faculty underscored the importance of knowing not only Alice's physiological state in order to be a competent practitioner and to pass boards, but also to listen to the heart of the patient's concern.

In another example, on the first day of class, an experienced faculty member invited graduate students to an online nursing theory course to write a nursing situation. A definition of a nursing situation and guidelines for writing were posted to help the students recapture the experience of caring between the nurse and the one nursed. Students shared their nursing situations with the faculty and fellow students. If a student posted a case study—a story about diagnosis and treatment—the story was revised and refined with faculty input to uncover and shine a light on the caring between nurse and nursed. The faculty member stated that she "wants the students to begin with a nursing situation so the course content has relevancy to their practice." She added, "Posting their nursing situations for all to read provides the milieu of shared values and respect for each other as they create a type of sisterhood and brotherhood of nursing in the course." Students reported this learning activity reawakened their love for nursing and rediscovery of the beauty in practice.

Similarly, a graduate course on evidence-based practice (EBP) and research was taught from the lens of nursing situations. Students were invited to write a nursing situation to use as an inspiration to develop a study question. Using the PICOT (population, intervention, comparison, outcome, and time) format, questions were used to structure a focused review of the literature and the development of an evidence-based practice question (Melnyk & Fineout-Overholt, 2010). The faculty stated: "Using nursing situations to develop these studies refines the general intention of EBP as a medical process into a process of nursing focused on understanding individuals in the context of a health experience."

The specific advanced practice courses of a curriculum are taught from the perspective of the Willow family, a fictitious family created by the faculty.

The faculty describes using the nursing situations of the Willow family to bring complex concepts to life for the students. The Willows experience the usual and sometimes unusual complexities of a contemporary family. Students embrace the family and its unfolding, as they study advanced practice in nursing situations related to pregnancy, birth, health and illness, relationships, growth, job loss, relocations, members moving in and out, aging, and death.

Nursing situations are described by another faculty member to guide the study of health care policy in a doctoral course. The students are asked to reflect on a nursing situation near and dear to their hearts that had an implication for policy change. One student described working in an intensive care unit (ICU) that had restricted visiting hours, despite all the research findings on the benefit of open visiting hours. She went on to describe how painful and sad it was for her patient and his wife, who came to visit during her lunch hour but was not allowed because of visiting hour restrictions. Just as she was about to enter the unit, doctors started making rounds and she was told she could not enter when rounds were taking place. She waited as long as she could to visit her husband but had to leave to return to work, and did not see him. The student identified compassion and courage as the essence of caring in this situation. The student spent the semester working on effecting a policy change for visiting hours based on the beneficial evidence to support a revised policy.

Chapter 5 provides a full description of teaching/learning using nursing situations in a graduate course focusing on the discipline of nursing.

MULTIPLE APPROACHES TO UNDERSTANDING CARING IN NURSING

A. Boykin (personal communication, April 10, 2014) states: "There is no predetermined nursing. The study of nursing situations evokes a unique understanding for both the faculty and student of the artistry of nursing practice and how each may experience the caring between in a different way. The intentional appreciation of the differences in apprehending the caring essence of a nursing situation contributes to the beauty of practice." This idea of the individual appreciation can be experienced in reflecting on the exemplars provided earlier. Although, both faculty and students had identified essential caring components in the nursing situations, re-presentation invites readers to experience the nursing situations anew and discover their own unique expressions of caring.

Mayeroff's (1971) philosophical work on caring in teaching is very useful for nursing. His thesis, "to be human is to be caring," has multidisciplinary appeal and rings particularly true for nursing. The eight caring ingredients—knowing, honesty, humility, alternating rhythms, trust, hope, courage, and patience—give immediate voice to nurses struggling to describe their nursing practice. Likewise Roach's (1987/2002) six Cs—compassion, commitment, conscience, comportment, competence, and confidence—developed for nursing practice have an immediate heuristic appeal to nurses and students of nursing and provide an "a-ha" moment of "Yes, that's what went on between my patient and myself today." Roach's work also draws nurses and students of nursing into a purposeful practice of reflection intent on understanding self and other as living caring the best as it can be in a particular moment.

The caring concepts of Mayeroff (1971) and Roach (1992) offer a basis of understanding caring in nursing, but there are others. Paterson and Zderad's (1988) description of presence is well described; and Boykin and Schoenhofer (2001) further conceptualize presence as authentic presence. In addition, Kolcaba's ideas on comfort (2010), Purnell's on intentionality (2002), Dunn and Riva's conception of compassion energy (2014), and Erikson's concept of love (1994) are examples of concepts that capture a unique experience of caring in nursing situations. But there may be others identified and conceptualized as teachers and students capture and identify meaningful expressions of caring. Chapter 2 presents a fuller description of caring in nursing.

MULTIPLE THEORETICAL APPROACHES TO STUDY NURSING SITUATIONS

The authors' approach to the study of nursing situations is from a particular lens of caring in nursing grounded in the philosophy of the Christine E. Lynn College of Nursing. Nursing is "nurturing the wholeness and well-being of persons and environment in caring" (FAU, CON, 2012, para. 1). The authors, however, acknowledge the usefulness of various theoretical approaches to study nursing from nursing situations.

Chapter 4 presents a comparison of guiding questions from the Barry, Gordon, and King (2013) Teaching/Learning Nursing Framework, with guiding questions adapted to several nursing theoretical perspectives that are commonly used in schools of nursing and practice settings. The language of selected theories is translated into language suitable for the analysis of nursing situations highlighting focused outcomes for the one nursed, the nurse, the nursing profession, and others in a rippling effect of meaning. The grand theories are Nursing as Caring (Boykin & Schoenhofer, 2001); Human Caring (Watson, 2010), Self-Care Deficit (Orem, 2006), The Theory of Culture Care Diversity and Universality (Leininger & McFarland, 2010); and the Roy Adaptation Model (Roy & Zahn, 2010). The two middle range theories included and compared for application to nursing situations are the theories of uncertainty in illness (Mishel & Clayton, 2008) and comfort theory (Kolcaba, 2010).

LANGUAGE

This book is written in a distinctive manner that focuses on the nurse and the one nursed. The words "client" and "patient" have been avoided unless they appear as a direct quote from a description of a nursing situation. Buber's philosophical work *I and Thou* (1958) has served as a foundation for many contemporary theories of nursing and serves as grounding for the respectful language of this text. In a translation of Buber's work, Stiles (2011) relates the caring between the nurse and the one nursed as a sacred space in which each beholds the other as Thou. This view of the other as Thou is the inspiration for the authors to write this text intentionally free of language that expresses or implies bias, disrespect, or prejudicial preferences for the other.

The notion of respectful language has been specifically promulgated by scholars of nursing and the American Psychological Association publication manual (American Psychological Association, 2009), and yet language that objectifies others and puts them in a box that limits our understanding is commonly heard, read, and used. This is not the situation with children with disabilities. Respectful language was introduced as an essential component of the Individuals With Disabilities Act (Family to Family Network, 2013). IDEA is known as the "person-first" law, recognizing the child first and disability second. The law forever changed language from handicapped children to children with disabilities, focusing attention on the individual and not on a condition or label.

Hills and Watson (2011) assert, "Caring Science, ethically and philosophically, seeks to avoid reducing any human, whether student or patient, or any other, to the moral status of object." (p. 12).

Once a person becomes an object, like a DNR (do not resuscitate) medical order, we as nurses can separate ourselves from the humanity of the other and in doing so lose some of our own humanity (Purnell, 2001). Buber calls us to experience the other as a human being; through this connection and interrelationship, we experience a fuller understanding of ourselves as human beings and as nurses.

Nursing situations are the touchstone and heart of this text, focusing on persons as individuals and not as cases of illness or disease such as "the diabetic patient" or "the DNR." In all instances, persons will be described as the individual with diabetes or the person with a DNR order or the individual with Alzheimer's disease. The authors envision a future in which nursing language always places the focus on the individual rather than the health concern.

SUMMARY

This chapter introduces the notion of nursing situations—contextualized stories from the day-to-day practice of nursing—as a repository of nursing knowledge and an innovative approach to teaching/learning nursing. This approach is developed in response to a call from national leaders and scholars to transform nursing education using methods that illuminate and unify the complexity of contemporary nursing practice. The tenets of narrative pedagogy provide the basis for this innovative approach and exemplars of teaching undergraduate and graduate students are offered. Various philosophical and theoretical approaches to nursing are presented as frameworks to examine nursing situations for knowledge and meaning. The authors conclude with a description of the use of specific language in this book that focuses on persons being cared for and not on the individual's heath concern.

REFERENCES

American Association of Colleges of Nursing (AACN). (2010). *The Essentials of baccalaureate education for professional nursing practice.* Washington, DC: Author.

American Psychological Association. (2010). *Publication manual of the American Psychological Association* (6th ed.). Washington, DC: Author.

Barry, C. (1990, April). *I am nurse.* Paper presented at the meeting of the International Association for Human Caring, Houston, TX.

Barry, C. D., Gordon, S. C., & King, B. (2013). Nursing situations: Teaching, learning and living caring in nursing [Abstract]. *International Journal for Human Caring, 17*(3), 50–51.

Benner, P., Sulphen, M., Leonard, V., & Day, L. (2010). *Educating nurses: A call for radical transformation.* San Francisco, CA: Jossey-Bass.

Boykin, A., & Schoenhofer, S. (2001). *Nursing as caring.* Boston, MA: Jones & Bartlett Publishers.

Buber, M. (1958). *I and thou* (2nd ed.). New York, NY: Charles Scribner's Sons.

The Carnegie Foundation for the Advancement of Teaching. (2010). *Book highlights from educating nurses: A call for radical transformation.* Retrieved from http://www.carnegiefoundation.org/elibrary/education-nures-highlights

Carper, B. (1978). Fundamental patterns of knowing in nursing. *Advances in Nursing Science, 1*(1), 13–24.

Chinn, P. L. (2014). Educating for social justice. *Journal of Nursing Education, 53*(9), 487.

Dunn, D. J., & Rivas, D. (2014). Transforming compassion satisfaction. *International Journal for Human Caring, 18*(1), 45–49.

Eriksson, K. (1994). Theories of caring as health. In D. Gaut & A. Boykin (Eds.), *Caring as healing: Renewal through hope* (pp. 3–20). New York, NY: National League for Nursing Press.

Family to Family Network. (2013). Retrieved from http://www.familytofamily network.org/parent-resources/people-first-language

Florida Atlantic University, Christine E. Lynn College of Nursing. (2012). *Philosophy.* Retrieved from http://nursing.fau.edu/index.php?main=1&nav=635

Hills, M., & Watson, J. (2011). *Creating a caring science curriculum: An emancipatory pedagogy for nursing.* New York, NY: Springer Publishing.

Institute of Medicine. (2011). *The future of nursing: Leading change, advancing health.* Washington, DC: Author.

The Joint Commission. (2014). *National patient safety goals 2014.* Retrieved from http://www.jointcommission.org/standards_information/npsgs.aspx

Kagen, P. N., Smith, M. C., Cowling, R., & Chinn, P. (2009). A nursing manifesto: An emancipatory call for nursing knowledge development, conscience, and practice. *Nursing Philosophy, 11*(1), 67–84.

King, B., Barry, C. D., & Gordon, S. C. (2014). Nursing situations: Teaching, learning and living caring in nursing [Abstract]. *International Journal for Human Caring, 17*(3), 50–51.

Kolcaba, K. (2010). Katherine Kolcaba's comfort theory. In M. Parker & M. Smith (Eds.), *Nursing theory and nursing practice* (3rd ed., pp. 389–401). Philadelphia, PA: F.A. Davis.

Leininger, M., & McFarland, M. R. (2010). The theory of culture care diversity and universality. In M. Parker & M. Smith (Eds.), *Nursing theory and nursing practice* (3rd ed., pp. 317–336). Philadelphia, PA: F.A. Davis.

Mayeroff, M. (1971). *On caring*. New York, NY: Harper & Row.

Melnyk, B. M., & Fineout-Overholt, E. (2010). *Evidence-based practice in nursing & healthcare: A guide to best practice*. Philadelphia, PA: Wolters Kluwer/Lippincott Williams & Wilkins.

Mishel, M. H., & Clayton, M. F. (2008). Theories of uncertainty in illness. In M. J. Smith & P. R. Liehr (Eds.), *Middle range theory for nursing* (2nd ed., pp. 55–84). New York, NY: Springer.

National League for Nursing (NLN). (2005). *Core competencies of nurse educators with tasks statements*. Retrieved from http://www.nln.org/profdev/corecompeten-cies.pdf

National Organization of Nurses Practitioner Faculty (NONPF). (2011). *Nurse practitioner core competencies*. Washington, DC: Author.

Newman, M. A., Sime, A. M., & Corcoran-Perry, S. A. (1991). The focus of the discipline of nursing. *Advances in Nursing Science, 14*(1), 1–6.

Orem, D. (2006). Dorothea E. Orem's self-care nursing theory. In M. Parker & M. Smith (Eds.), *Nursing theory and nursing practice* (2nd ed., pp. 144–149). Philadelphia, PA: F.A. Davis.

Paterson, J., & Zderad, L. (1988). *Humanistic nursing*. New York, NY: National League for Nursing Press.

Purnell, M. J. (2001). The language of nursing: A technology of caring. In R. Locsin (Ed.), *Advancing technology, caring, and nursing* (pp. 53–67). Westport, CT: Auburn.

Purnell, M. J. (2002). Issue editor. Why nurses nurse! Intentionality in Nursing. *Holistic Nursing Practice, 16*(4), vi–ix.

Quality Safety Education in Nursing. (2005). *Press release phase I*. Retrieved from http://qsen.org/about-qsen/project-overview/project-phases/

Roach, M. S. (1992). *The human act of caring*. Ottawa, Canada: Canadian Hospital Association.

Roach, M. S. (1987/2002). *Caring, the human mode of being: A blueprint for the health professions (2nd rev. ed)*. Ottawa, Canada: The Canadian Hospital Association Press.

Roy, C., & Zahn, L. (2010). Sister Callista Roy's adaptation model. In M. Parker & M. Smith (Eds.), *Nursing theory and nursing practice* (3rd ed., pp. 167–181). Philadelphia, PA: F.A. Davis.

Smith, M. C. (2013). Caring and the discipline of nursing. In M. Smith, M. Turkey, & Z. Wolf (Eds.), *Caring in nursing classics* (pp. 1–8). New York, NY: Springer Publishing.

Stiles, K. A. (2011). Advancing nursing knowledge through complex holism. *Advances in Nursing Science, 44*(1), 39–50.

Sullivan, W. (2008). *A new agenda for higher education: Shaping a life of the mind for practice*. San Francisco, CA: Jossey-Bass.

Swanson, K. (1991). Empirical development of a middle-range theory. *Nursing Research, 40*(3), 161–166.

Touhy, T., & Boykin, A. (2008). Caring as the central domain in nursing. *International Journal for Human Caring, 12*(2), 9–15.

U.S. Department of Health and Human Services. (2014). Healthy People 2020. Retrieved from http://www.healthypeople.gov/2020/about/default.aspx

Watson, J. (1979). *Nursing: The philosophy and science of caring*. Boston, MA: Little Brown.

Watson, J. (2010). Jean Watson's theory of human caring. In M. Parker & M. Smith (Eds.), *Nursing theory and nursing practice* (3rd ed., pp. 351–369). Philadelphia, PA: F. A. Davis.

Philosophical and Theoretical Perspectives of Caring, Knowing, and Story Underpinning the Study of Nursing Situations

The study of nursing through nursing situations is grounded in two basic assumptions: (a) The essence of nursing is caring, and (b) all nursing knowledge resides in nursing situations.

The purpose of Chapter 2 is to describe underpinnings of the caring nature of the discipline and practice of nursing, patterns of knowing in nursing, theories of narrative knowing, and the use of situated stories of professional practice supporting the process of teaching/learning from nursing situations as essential to the study and practice of nursing. These underpinnings are considered foundational to the use of stories or nursing situations in nursing education. Readers are encouraged to read widely on the topics that are only briefly considered in this chapter.

CARING NATURE OF THE DISCIPLINE AND PRACTICE OF NURSING: PHILOSOPHICAL AND THEORETICAL VIEWS

The purpose of this section is to describe major philosophical and theoretical views that have influenced the study of nursing as caring, caring science, and teaching from nursing situations. A theory is generally described as an idea or gathering of ideas that is useful in explaining a phenomenon of interest. The following are examples of definitions of theory commonly used in nursing:

- Theory is a set of ideas, concepts, definitions, and propositions that project a systematic view of phenomena by designating specific inter-relationships among concepts for purposes of describing, explaining, predicting, and/or controlling phenomena (Chinn & Jacobs, 1987, p. 71).
- A theory is an imaginative grouping of knowledge, ideas, and experience that are represented symbolically and seek to illuminate a given phenomenon (Watson, 1985, p. 1).

It is theory that helps us articulate how disciplines are distinct from one another. Theories are particularly useful in explicating the domain or focus of a discipline. For example, the focus of medicine is on the diagnosis and treatment of disease. Nursing assumes a multitheoretical focus in which each nursing theory posits a unique focus of nursing and provides guiding boundaries for practice, education, and research.

As described, theories are human inventions evaluated in terms of their usefulness to explain phenomena, interpret practice and research findings, enhance our knowing of nursing, predict outcomes, and raise important research questions. They define and are part of the knowledge structure of the discipline.

Theoretical knowledge structure is reflected in levels of theoretical development. Theories vary in the level of abstraction in which phenomena of interest to the discipline are described. Theories of the middle range were originally defined by Merton (1968) as broad enough to be useful in complex situations and appropriate for empirical testing. Smith and Liehr (2008) suggest that because middle range theories have a narrower scope than grand theories, they may be more effective in increasing theory-based research and nursing practice intervention. Comfort Theory (Kolcaba, 2010) and Theory of Uncertainty in Illness (Mishel, 1988) are examples of middle range theories presented in Chapter 4.

Practice level theories are the least abstract and have a limited scope. They are developed within the context of a specific range of nursing situations. Nurses, students, educators, and researchers are drawn to theories of the middle range and practice level because they closely represent day-to-day nursing experiences and are the most applicable to nursing practice. Practice theories are interdependent with middle range and/or grand theories. Watson and Foster's (2003) attendant nurse caring model is an example of a practice level theory.

PHILOSOPHICAL AND THEORETICAL THEORIES OF CARING

Scholars Mayeroff (1971) and Roach (2002) have identified major ingredients and attributes of caring. Building in part on these early descriptions of caring, Paterson and Zderad (1988), Boykin and Schoenhofer (2001), and

Watson (1985) have asserted philosophical and theoretical views of caring linked to the use of nursing situations to study nursing. The following sections provide a brief overview of these significant works.

In 1971, Mayeroff published a book with the intent to explore the concepts of "caring" and the relationship of care to a sense of being "in place" in the world. He defined caring as a process of helping "another to grow and actualize himself" (p. 1). The basic thesis of this work was "through caring for certain others, by serving them through caring, a man lives the meaning of his life" (p. 2). He affirmed that by relating to others through caring, persons live their own values and beliefs authentically and are at home in the world. Mayeroff's major ingredients of caring (knowing, alternating rhythms, patience, honesty, trust, humanity, hope, and courage) were offered to a general audience; however, they are useful in understanding caring in nursing.

Mayeroff challenged the common idea that caring does not require knowledge. He discussed the importance of knowing "many things," both general and specific, as necessary to support caring. From his perspective, caring requires understanding who the other is, what his or her needs are, what is conducive to the other's growth, what the other's powers and limitations are, how to respond properly to needs, and to understand powers and limitations of self (p. 19).

Alternating rhythm, "the rhythm of moving back and forth between a narrower and wider framework" (p. 32), was identified as the caring ingredient required to consider an event or idea in isolation and in a wider context of what has gone before. From a nursing perspective, alternating rhythms allow us to focus on a specific event or behavior while continuing to see the person in the context of wholeness. For example, nurses may focus on a person's individual act of self-injury, while moving to a wider framework to consider past patterns of behavior as well as personal strengths and support networks.

Caring as an expression of belief in the growth of others requires patience. Patience "enables the other to grow in its own time and in its own way" (p. 23). Giving time to the other through patience requires an active participation and constitutes a gift of self. An impatient encounter diminishes the time and space the other has to learn, feel, and grow. Caring is demonstrated in nursing when nurses patiently listen to someone tell his or her story, tolerate a certain amount of uncertainty by providing needed time and space, and offer support as persons nursed discover the meaning of a health-related event in the context of their lives. Mayeroff also encourages patience with self to "give myself a chance to care," learn, and grow (p. 24).

Genuinely caring for another requires honesty with self and others. Barriers to caring are created when there are gaps between how one honestly feels and acts. In other words, one cannot pretend to care. Helping the other to grow (to care) requires seeing the other as he or she is, not as one would like him or her to be. This understanding is necessary in hearing and developing meaningful nursing calls and responses. Honesty also requires the evaluation of nursing responses to determine if they are helping or diminishing growth.

"Caring involves trusting the other to grow in its own time and in its own way" (p. 27). Not trusting in the other results in unresponsiveness to the needs of the other. However, trust is not passive. It is grounded in actively promoting the growth of others and safeguarding the other in conditions as warranted. For example, when caring for a person who recently began insulin injections, the nurse demonstrates trust while actively assisting and encouraging the other as he or she learns to determine correct dosages and perform auto-injections safely. By trusting in the ability of the other to care for self, the nurse helps the other to grow.

Humility requires being willing to learn about the other person and self in order to understand the needs of the other and help him or her to grow. It requires being open to learn from any source, including learning from the mistakes. The belief that there is nothing to learn from someone else, or that one's caring is more important than the caring of others, is the antithesis of humility (Mayeroff, 1971).

Hope brings forth a present that is "alive with possibilities," "rallies energies," and "activates our powers" (p. 33). Hoping the other will grow in response to caring is not passive. It requires "standing up for the other in trying circumstances" (p. 33). The nurse intentionally enters each nursing situation with hope for something better in the moment. Hope requires the nurse to remain open to the possibilities for the other to grow in ways that are meaningful to the individual, family, or group. Hope is not possible without courage.

Courage is required to enter the world of the other. Courage to go into the unknown comes from trusting the other to grow as well as trusting in one's own ability to care (p. 34). As the nurse enters into a nursing situation, she or he cannot predict what the outcomes will be. However, nursing situations are not entered into blindly. Past knowledge and experience provide insight and guidance while the nurse maintains an openness to the present and future.

This book is grounded in the belief that caring is the essence of nursing. Caring, defined by Mayeroff as "helping the other to grow," is rooted in the service of helping others. His caring ingredients offer insight and meaning into the co-creation of caring relationships in nursing.

Roach (2002) offers a language of essential attributes of caring. She identifies attributes of caring—known as the Six Cs—that are intended as functional and ethical manifestations of professional caring. They are: compassion, competence, confidence, conscience, commitment, and comportment.

Compassion is defined as "a way of living born out of an awareness of one's relationship to all living creatures" (p. 50). This awareness invites participation in the experience of another, a sensitivity to another's pain and brokenness, and a quality of presence that allows making room for sharing with another. Compassion is an indispensable attribute of the caring relationship because it allows one to be fully immersed in the condition of being human. However, compassion without competence is not sufficient to meet the human care requirements of another.

Competence is defined by Roach as "the state of having the knowledge, judgments, skills, energy, experience, and motivation required to respond adequately to the demands of one's professional responsibility" (p. 54). Professional caring, such as caring in nursing, demands competence. However, Roach cautions that the misuse of power is a threat to caring competence and invites reflection on "competence as caring" versus "competence as manipulation" as nurses enter into caring relationships. Roach warns competence without compassion and humility can be an expression of brutality.

Confidence is "the quality which fosters trusting relationships" (p. 56). Confidence is required to create conditions of mutual trust and respect between the nurse and one nursed. The one nursed demonstrates respect for the nurse and has confidence in the nurse's willingness and ability to understand calls and respond in ways that are meaningful. It is in this co-created environment of mutual trust that professional caring relationships emerge.

Conscience is "understood as the morally sensitive self attuned to values" (p. 58). Caring conscience is an expression of responding to something that matters. It is "the call of care and manifests itself as care" (Heidegger, as cited in Roach, p. 61). Professional caring requires an understanding of the moral complexities of human relationships and a mature conscience built upon experience, moral inquiry, and knowledge of the discipline.

Commitment, defined as "a complex affective response characterized by a convergence between one's desires and one's obligations, and by a deliberate choice to act in accordance with them" (p. 62), is experienced at different levels at different times in professional caring. In a practice sense, professional caring requires a convergence of what one wants to do and what should be done (p. 62). It is an ongoing call to intentional, positive action. However, actions vary in the level of reflection required. The more difficult the choice, the more deliberate reflection is needed. Roach warns us that without commitment, "caring breaks down" (p. 62).

Comportment is reflected in demeanor and bearing. Therefore, professional comportment requires a harmony between language, dress, and caring image. Presenting a caring image of self by intentionally selecting language and dress that reflects a respectful attitude toward self, persons, or events is an expression of professional comportment.

For Roach, professional caring is expressed through human behaviors that include: "compassionate and competent acts; in relationships qualified by confidence, through informed sensitive conscience; and through commitment and fidelity" (p. 66). She challenges all of us to identify explicit caring acts in our day-to-day nursing practice by reflecting on the ontological questions:

- How does one want to live?
- What obligations are entailed in particular choices?
- What constitutes caring in everyday life of a professional person?
- What is a person doing when he or she is caring? (p. 66)

In addition to explications of caring ingredients (Mayeroff, 1971) and attributes of professional caring (Roach, 2002), several nurse scholars have asserted theoretical views of caring. The theories of Paterson and Zderad (1988), Boykin and Schoenhofer (2001), and Watson (1985) significantly influenced the development of the framework used in this text to support the study of nursing through the use of nursing situations. The footprints of these theorists can be seen in the King, Barry, and Gordon (2014) framework and are briefly described in the next few paragraphs.

In the process of searching for a way to improve the practice of nursing for nurses and ones nursed, Paterson and Zderad (1988) developed "humanistic nursing theory." The theorists were particularly interested in capturing the importance of day-to-day nursing activities, which they viewed from an existential lens of "being in the world." Important elements of their work include the concepts being, becoming, and change. For Paterson and Zderad, the purpose of nursing is "nurturing the well-being or more-being of persons in need" (p. 4). This focus affirms the "all-at-once" nature of nursing.

The concepts of call and response are integral to Paterson and Zderad's theory. Nursing begins with a call for help with a health-related concern. The call may come from an individual, community, or humanity. The nurse, upon hearing and recognizing the call, responds with intention to help. From the perspective of humanistic nursing, nursing happens in between the call and response—which they call *the between*. Paterson and Zderad offered phenomenological inquiry as the method for exploring the between. Phenomenological reflection on experiences refers to the process nurses use to bring forward the values and meanings present in their lived experiences to share with other nurses. Their writings lead the way for the development of future existential, phenomenological, and caring conceptualizations of nursing theory.

Watson's (1985) Theory of Human Caring is perhaps the best known theory of caring guiding nursing practice, research, and education. Major conceptual elements of her theory include 10 carative factors, transpersonal caring relationships, caring moments, and caring-healing modalities (Watson & Woodard, 2010, p. 353). Recently, Watson has reframed carative factors as "caritas processes" and "clinical caritas." The concept "caritas" connotes love and "allows love and caring to come together to form deep transpersonal caring" (p. 353) and the creation of caring moments through the use of caring–healing modalities. For Watson, transpersonal caring relationships move beyond ego self to connect with spiritual concerns that allow the nurse to access healing possibilities and potentials (p. 356). It is her belief that the one caring and the one being cared for are interconnected in a transpersonal caring relationship and the whole caring–healing consciousness is contained within a single caring–healing moment (p. 358). From this perspective, the focus of nursing is the transpersonal caring relationship between the nurse and the ones being cared for that creates harmony, wholeness, and unity of being in caring moments. From the perspective of this book, caring–healing moments take place within nursing situations.

Building upon the existential work of Paterson and Zderad (1988), Roach (2002), Mayeroff (1971), and curriculum development in the College of Nursing at Florida Atlantic University, Boykin and Schoenhofer (2001) developed the theory of nursing as caring as an organizing framework for nursing. The main assumption of the theory work is drawn from Roach's (2002) thesis that "caring is the human mode of being" (p. 7). The formative ideas of "call and response," "nursing response," and "personhood" form the structural basis for the theory. In addition, Mayeroff's caring ingredients were incorporated to provide the practical language of caring in nursing situations. Caring is defined as an "altruistic, active expression of love and is the intentional and embodied recognition of value and connectedness" (Boykin, Schoenhofer, & Linden, 2010, p. 372). However, the theorists caution the full meaning of caring cannot be expressed in a conceptual definition.

They defined the term "nursing situation" as "a shared lived experience in which the caring between nurse and nursed enhances personhood" (p. 372). They assert it is in the "in between" (p. 372) that caring is lived between the nurse and the one nursed. They assert "the practical knowledge of nursing lives within the context of person-to-person caring" (2010, p. 372). This statement supports a major theme of this book: "The use of nursing situations or narratives from practice, that illuminate the caring between the nurse and the one nursed inspire a heuristic approach to teaching/learning" (King, Barry, & Gordon, in review, p. 4).

KNOWING AND STORY UNDERPINNING THE STUDY OF NURSING SITUATIONS

Knowing in nursing is essential to the study and practice of nursing and is foundational to the use of case studies, stories, or nursing situations in nursing education. Based on their unique focus, members of a discipline determine the types of knowledge that are needed and the ways in which knowledge is developed, structured, and shared. Knowledge development, critique, dissemination, and application can be conceptualized as part of the dialogue of the discipline.

PATTERNS OF KNOWING IN NURSING

Patterns of knowing provide an overall structure for the knowledge of the discipline. Structuring nursing knowledge enhances our understanding of the depth and breadth of the unique body of nursing knowledge: what we know and what gaps exist in the extant literature. This understanding illuminates needed areas of research and guides the design and evaluation of nursing curricula.

Patterns of knowing, described by Carper (1978), and expanded upon by Boykin and Schoenhofer (1993), Munhall (1993), White (1995), and Kagen, Smith, Cowling, and Chinn (2009), assist us in knowing what to think about when thinking about nursing in the context of nursing situations. They serve "as a framework for asking epistemological questions of caring in nursing" (Boykin & Schoenhofer, 2001, p. 42). The structure of nursing knowledge is foundational to the use of stories of nursing situations in nursing education. Examples of epistemological questions from grand and middle range theories are provided in Chapter 4.

Historically, the journey toward developing a knowledge structure that truly reflects the unique perspective of nursing has been controversial. Prior to the development of nursing theories, the knowledge of nursing was primarily drawn from other related disciplines such as medicine, biology, and psychology combined with traditions of caring.

Carper (1978) was one of the first nursing scholars to address structuring nursing knowledge from a research perspective. Her work was revolutionary in its time and challenged nurses to think differently about traditional ways of approaching teaching/learning nursing. She theorized, "the body of nursing knowledge that serves as the rationale for nursing practice has patterns...that serve as organizing principles" (p. 13).

Carper used Phenix's 1964 model of "distinguishing types of meaning" (Carper, 1978, p. 14) to guide a review of the nursing literature from which she identified four categories she termed patterns of knowing: "(a) empirics, the science of knowing; (b) esthetics, the art of nursing; (c) the component of personal knowledge in nursing; and (d) ethics, the component of moral knowledge" (Carper, 1978, p. 14).

The first fundamental pattern of knowing is empirics, the science of knowing. It is generally described as "nursing science" (p. 19) and involves identifying, synthesizing, and applying scientific evidence to guide the practice of nursing. Disciplinary knowledge is developed in stages beginning with pre-paradigm conceptual structures and theoretical models that present new or expanded conceptualizations of phenomena. The next stage is "deductively formulated theory" (p. 20) involving description and classification of phenomena of interest to the discipline that leads to testing and verification of knowledge. Empirics or nursing science is the most understood and best described pattern of knowing in the nursing literature.

Esthetics, described by Carper as the art of nursing, acknowledges an understanding of nursing as both a science and an art. Early explications refer to esthetics as the artful performance of technical skills in the practice of nursing. Carper expanded the concept to incorporate art as an expressive pattern of knowing involving both creation and appreciation in which the art of nursing is visualized in the creation of nursing actions that reflect the needs of patients. Carper saw empathy as an important mode in coming to know the patient in the context of a "unique particular" rather than an "abstracted universal" (p. 22). She cautioned that without empathy and consideration of the patient as a unique, integrated whole, nursing actions may become a "mechanical routine" (p. 22) leading to dehumanized care.

Carper identified personal knowledge as "essential to understanding the meaning of health in terms of individual well-being" (p. 23). "Personal knowing is concerned with the knowing, encountering, and actualization of the concrete, individual self" (p. 23). Knowing self is a necessary element of being able to respond to patients with a therapeutic use of self. Therapeutic use of self involves entering into an authentic interpersonal relationship in which the patient is recognized as being in a constant state of growth. Through personal knowing, nurses engage persons and promote wholeness and integrity.

Nurses face difficult personal choices day-to-day in the context of complex, rapidly changing health care systems. Carper presented ethics, the moral component of nursing, as being focused on personal and professional obligations and "what ought to be done." Ethical knowing emerges from an examination of the beliefs, codes, and standards of the profession of nursing. However, it goes beyond simply knowing the ethical norms embedded in standards and codes. Ethical knowing encompasses all voluntary actions by the nurse that are deliberate and subject to judgment (either right or wrong) in relation to the individual nurse's intention and motive. Nurses must consider "what is good, what is right" (p. 21) from the perspective of different ethical frameworks and a full understanding of professional obligation.

All of the patterns of knowing are necessary, but none of the patterns are sufficient on their own to guide nursing practice, research, and education. Carper's patterns of knowing offer an increased awareness of the importance of structuring nursing knowledge. Patterns of knowing draw "attention to the question of what it means to know and what kinds of knowledge are held to be of most value in the discipline of nursing" (p. 13).

Over time, scholars have critiqued and expanded Carper's work. In 1993, Boykin, Parker, and Schoenhofer critiqued Carper's original work. They asserted Carper did not (a) ground her description of aesthetics explicitly in a conception of nursing, (b) distinguish clearly between knowledge and knowing, or (c) fully describe the role of the aesthetic pattern of knowing in nursing. In response, the authors proposed "a new understanding of aesthetic knowing in nursing, grounded in an explicit conception of nursing" (p. 158).

Grounded in the theory of Nursing as Caring, Boykin and Schoenhofer (1993) described an expanded conceptualization of aesthetic knowing as an "integrative nursing way of knowing" (p. 160) "essential to understanding and doing nursing" (p. 159). "Aesthetic knowing in nursing is the creating experience in the nursing situation, the expression of the experience, and appreciation of it through encounter" (p. 158). The authors assert that through the aesthetic way of knowing, the art of nursing is "appreciated, known and studied" (p. 161). They described aesthetic knowing as necessary in bringing "empirical, ethical, and personal knowing to the situation" (p. 161). Through aesthetic knowing, a "full realization of the interconnection of persons and objects" is understood (p. 160). Nursing is affirmed as an *unfolding process* in which "the result of nursing cannot be foreseen" rather than as a specific product or outcome (p. 161).

In 1993, Munhall added a fifth pattern of knowing that she called "unknowing." She explored unknowing as a condition of openness that serves as a necessary precursor of coming to know the other. The art of unknowing enables the nurse to understand, with empathy, the actual essence of the meaning an experience has for a patient. Unknowing requires the nurse to be open to learning the needs of another, or to truly hear a colleague, a teacher, or a student. To provide and find openness is to be able to think about experiences in new ways and encounter the wonderment of coming upon an *unknown*. When you are open to unknowing, you are open to learning things "you never knew you never knew" (Menken & Swartz, 1995). A nurse who cares wants to truly know the other. The nurse intentionally sets aside his or her knowingness to be open to learning what the other is experiencing.

White (1995) expanded Carper's patterns of knowing to include sociopolitical knowing, which was designed to move the focus of knowing away from the patient and nurse to address the broader context in which nursing and health care takes place—which they called the *wherein*. White conceptualized sociopolitical knowing as involving the context of persons (nurse–patient relationships) and nursing as a practice profession (society and politics). She described the context of persons as including culture, meanings attached to health and disease, and language. For White, this pattern of knowing also addresses historical issues such as connection and dislocation from land and heritage (p. 84).

Nursing takes place in the context of society and politics that influence both patient conditions and nursing roles. For example, Chopoorian (1986) suggested, "Nursing practitioners continually confront the human responses to the underlying social dynamics of poverty, unemployment, undernutrition, isolation, and alienation precipitated through the structures of society" (pp. 40–41). Many of the problems nurses see affecting others are the result of fundamentally social rather than personal problems. Examples include limited access to health care, violence, drug abuse, and chronic illnesses such as diabetes and asthma. Sociopolitical knowing obligates nurses to address underlying social structures contributing to patient conditions or outcomes through advocacy strategies such as sharing what they see and know with policy makers and participating in decision-making processes.

More recently, Purnell (2009) challenged nurses to move away from applying Carper's patterns of knowing in a linear fashion and explore knowing in nursing more fully. She argued that Carper's four patterns of knowing, as often presented and applied, are not sufficient to study the fullness of nursing or for nursing scholars to describe knowing of nursing and address the many phenomena of interest to the discipline. Purnell argued integration of knowing, necessary for nursing practice, was missing from Carper's presentation of patterns of knowing as distinct and separate patterns.

In response, Purnell revisited Phenix's (1964) symbolic and synoptic realms and corresponding patterns of meaning. Symbolic meaning was described by Phenix as the most basic pattern of meaning. Simply put, symbolic meaning refers to the meanings we attach to everyday concepts. For example, an elementary school health room might evoke images of safety for young students. Therefore, the symbolic meaning of the concept *school room* may be safety. Because language is a form of symbolic expression, it is through symbolic meaning that we come to understand and express our understanding of all other patterns of meaning. Aesthetic expression is also useful when language is insufficient to fully express knowing; for example, describing the grief nurses bear witness to when parents suffer the loss of a child.

Phenix termed the realm in which meaning from all realms are comprehensively integrative as the *synoptic realm* (1964, p. 7). Purnell interpreted Phenix's concepts of synoptic and symbolic realms of meaning as representing "two different expressions of the same knowing" (p. 13). She transferred the symbolic and synoptic realms into one unitary pattern of knowing in nursing, conceptualized as "synoptic or integrative knowing in nursing practice" (p. 14). Synoptic knowing involves pulling together all that is known into a comprehensive, integrative whole. Purnell suggests it is synoptic knowing "that is the most at home within the nursing situation" (p. 12). Through synoptic knowing, nursing knowledge not yet known might be discovered.

Chinn and Kramer (2011) have also contributed to our understanding of ways of knowing in nursing. Like Purnell and Boykin and Schoenhofer, Chinn and Kramer asserted the need to address an integration of Carper's patterns of knowing into a unified whole. They extended Carper's work to include emancipatory knowing that they defined as a process of understanding barriers that create unfair and unjust social conditions that motivate action to improve people's lives (p. 248). Emancipatory knowing lived as a nursing practice with and for people served reflects nursing art and science as an integration of multiple patterns of knowing that are useful in guiding knowledge development, education, and practice.

NARRATIVE KNOWING AND USE OF SITUATED STORIES OF PROFESSIONAL PRACTICE

In 2009, Benner, Sulphen, Leonard, and Day identified the need for teaching strategies that encourage students to focus on the human experience in the context of individual patients and families in their landmark nursing education study, *Educating Nurses: A Call for Radical Transformation*. They asserted the focus on the human experience was essential in facilitating the student's clinical reasoning ability and encouraged the use of multiple ways of thinking. The Institute of Medicine (2011) report, *The Future of Nursing: Leading Change, Advancing Health,* soon followed and echoed the need for new educational models designed to develop critical thinking, facilitate decision making, and develop competencies to meet the demanding, ever-changing world of health care.

Although the landmark reports described previously refer to the need for new educational models, nursing has a rich history of recognizing the importance of narrative knowing and the use of situated stories of professional practice to inform the study of the discipline. Theories of narrative knowing and use of situated stories of professional practice are discussed from the viewpoints of Coles (1989), Diekelmann (1990), and Sandelowski (1991).

Coles (1989), writing about his experiences as a student, physician, and educator, advanced the usefulness of the "call of story" in practice and education to come to know others and self and as a form of moral support. He suggested a reconceptualization of how health care providers approach coming to know patients. He described the value in listening for and to patient stories in place of focusing solely on obtaining a traditional clinical history. He reminds us: "The people who come to see us bring us their stories. They hope they tell them well enough so that we understand the truth of their lives" (p. 7). He encourages us to be open to the possibility of learning what happened within each story and to base what we are thinking about a patient on what he or she tells us. If we listen to the patient's stories we will learn from them what is hurting, what is happening in their lives, and what they think is wrong (p. 30). For Coles, respecting individual stories and learning from them is the moral imperative of "fellow humans in need" (p. 205). Through engaging in the intimacy of the shared stories of others, we also come to know ourselves as human beings and practitioners. We begin by inviting others (patients, students, and colleagues) to "just share a story or two" (p. 11).

Shared stories also form the basis of the teaching approach known as narrative pedagogy. Narrative pedagogy, described by Diekelmann in the 1990s, focuses on the lived experience through the use of narratives from practice (Diekelmann, 1990, 2001; Nehls, 1995). Diekelmann (2001) describes narrative pedagogy as a "gathering of all the pedagogies into converging conversation such that the possibility for anything to show itself is held open" (p. 55). Using this approach to the study of nursing, teachers and students collectively come together to study and learn from lived practice experiences shared as narratives. Thoughtful dialogue encourages the teacher and student to reflect together on the shared narrative from multiple perspectives. In the dialogue, theory and practice are linked and openness to the possibilities of nursing care is created.

Dialogue is essential to nursing education and the process of coming to know caring in the context of nursing practice. It requires "engaged listening, seeking to understand, and being open to all possibilities" (Diekelmann, 1990, p. 301). It moves us away from approaching nursing education from a strict pedagogy of behaviorism and grounds curricula and teaching methods in the day-to-day practice and clinical experiences of students and faculty.

Sharing recalled narratives from nursing practice allows others to be "drawn into and within" (Baker & Diekelmann, 1994, p. 66) the nurse's understandings and invites personal reflection. In the dialogue exploring presented narratives, participants recall stories from their own practice that have special meaning to them and share reflections on their understandings, values, and beliefs. In this way, "narratives can begin to create new understandings about the nature of content and thinking in education" (Diekelmann, 1993).

SUMMARY

This chapter presents the philosophical and theoretical perspectives of caring, knowing, and story underpinning the study of nursing situations. King, Barry, and Gordon (2014) share Boykin and Schoenhofer's (2001) assumption that "the knowledge of nursing resides in the nursing situation and is brought to life through study" (p. 42). The study of nursing situations defined as "co-created lived experiences in which the caring between the nurses and persons enhanced well-being" (FAU, CON, 2012) unfolds from philosophical and theoretical perspectives of caring, concepts of knowing, and the use of stories or narratives from nursing practice.

REFERENCES

Baker, C., & Diekelmann, N. (1994). Connecting conversations of caring: Recalling the narrative to clinical practice. *Nursing Outlook, 42*(2), 65–70.

Benner, P., Sulphen, M., Leonard, V., & Day, L. (2009). *Educating nurses: A call for radical transformation.* San Francisco, CA: Jossey-Bass.

Boykin, A., Parker, M. E., & Schoenhofer, S. O. (1993). Aesthetic knowing grounded in an explicit conception of nursing. *Nursing Science Quarterly, 7*(4), 158–161.

Boykin, A., & Schoenhofer, S. O. (1993). *Nursing as caring: A model for transforming practice.* New York, NY: National League for Nursing Press.

Boykin, A., & Schoenhofer, S. (2001). *Nursing as caring: A model for transforming practice.* Boston, MA: Jones & Bartlett Publishers.

Boykin, A., Schoenhofer, S., & Linden, D. (2010). Anne Boykin and Savina Schoenhofer's nursing as caring theory. In M. E. Parker & M. C. Smith (Eds.), *Nursing theories & nursing practice* (3rd ed., pp. 370–386). Philadelphia, PA: F.A. Davis.

Carper, B. (1978). Fundamental patterns of knowing in nursing. *Advances in Nursing Science, 1*(1), 13–23.

Chinn, P., & Jacobs, M. (1987). *Theory and nursing: A systematic approach.* St. Louis, MO: C.V. Mosby.

Chinn, P., & Kramer, M. (2011). *Integrated theory and knowledge development in nursing.* St. Louis, MO: Mosby/Elsevier.

Chopoorian, T. (1986). Reconceptualizing the environment. In P. Mocia (Ed.), *New approaches to theory development* (pp. 39–54). New York, NY: National League for Nursing Press.

Coles, R. (1989). *The call of stories.* Boston, MA: Houghton Mifflin.

Diekelmann, N. L. (1990). Nursing education: Caring, dialogue, and practice. *Journal of Nursing Education, 29*(7), 300–305.

Diekelmann, N. L. (1993). Behavioral pedagogy: A Heideggerian hermeneutical analysis of the lived experiences of students and teachers in baccalaureate nursing education. *Journal of Nursing Education, 32*(6), 245–250.

Diekelmann, N. L. (2001). Narrative pedagogy: Heideggerian hermeneutical analyses of lived experiences of students, teachers, and clinicians. *Advances in Nursing Science, 23*(3), 53–71.

Florida Atlantic University, Christine E. Lynn College of Nursing. (2012). *Philosophy.* Retrieved from http://nursing.fau.edu/index.php?main=1&nav=635

Institute of Medicine. (2011). *The future of nursing: Leading change, advancing health.* Washington, DC: The National Academies Press.

Kagen, P. N., Smith, M. C., Cowling, W. R., & Chinn, P. L. (2009). A manifesto: An emancipatory call for knowledge development, conscience, and praxis. *Nursing Philosophy, 11*, 67–84.

King, B., Barry, C., & Gordon, S. (2014). Lived experience of teaching/learning from nursing situations: A phenomenological study [Abstract]. *International Journal for Human Caring, 18*(3), 88.

King, B. M., Barry, C. D., & Gordon, S. C. (in review). The lived experience of teaching and learning from nursing situations: A phenomenological study. *Journal for Human Caring* (accepted for publication).

Kolcaba, K. (2010). Katherine Kolcaba's comfort theory. In M. E. Parker & M. C. Smith (Eds.), *Nursing theories and nursing practice* (3rd ed., pp. 389–401). Philadelphia, PA: F.A. Davis.

Mayeroff, M. (1971). *On caring.* New York, NY: Harper & Row.

Menken, A., & Swartz, S. L. (1995). *Colors of the wind.* Burbank, CA: Wonderland Music Company, Inc., and Walt Disney Music Company, Ltd. Retrieved from http://www.stlyrics.com/lyrics/classicdisney/colorsofthewind.htm

Merton, R. (1968). *Social theory and social structure.* New York, NY: The Free Press.

Mishel, M. H. (1988). Uncertainty in illness. *Image: Journal of Nursing Scholarship, 20*(4), 225–232.

Munhall, P. (1993). Unknowing: Toward another pattern of knowing. *Nursing Outlook, 41*, 125–128.

Nehls, N. (1995). Narrative pedagogy: Rethinking nursing education. *Journal of Nursing Education, 34*(5), 204–210.

Paterson, J., & Zderad, L. (1988). *Humanistic nursing.* New York, NY: National League for Nursing.

Phenix, P. H. (1964). *Realms of meaning: A philosophy of the curriculum for general education.* New York, NY: McGraw-Hill.

Purnell, M. J. (2009). Phoenix arising: Synoptic knowing for a synoptic practice of nursing. In R. C. Locsin & M. J. Purnell (Eds.), *A contemporary nursing process: The (un)bearable weight of knowing in nursing* (pp. 1–16). New York, NY: Springer.

Roach, M. S. (1987/2002). *Caring, the human mode of being: A blueprint for the health professions (2nd rev. ed)*. Ottawa, Canada: The Canadian Hospital Association Press.

Roach, M. S. (2002). *The human act of caring: A blueprint for the health professions*. Ottawa, Canada: The Canadian Hospital Association Press.

Sandelowski, M. (1991). Telling stories, narrative approaches in qualitative research. *Image: Journal of Nursing Scholarship, 23*(3), 163–166.

Smith, M. J., & Liehr, P. R. (2008). *Middle range theory for nursing* (2nd ed.). New York, NY: Springer.

Watson, J., & Foster, R. (2003). The attending nurse caring model: Integrating theory, evidence and advanced caring-healing therapeutics for transforming professional practice. *Journal of Clinical Nursing, 12*(3), 360–365.

Watson, J., & Woodward, T. K. (2010). Jean Watson's theory of human caring. In M. E. Parker & M. C. Smith (Eds.), *Nursing theories and nursing practice* (3rd ed., pp. 352–369). Philadelphia, PA: F.A. Davis.

Watson, J. (1985). *Nursing: Human science and human care*. Norwalk, CT: Appleton-Century-Crofts.

White, J. (1995). Patterns of knowing: Review, critique, and update. *Advances in Nursing Science, 17*(4), 73–86.

CHAPTER 3

Barry, Gordon & King Framework for Teaching/ Learning Nursing

This chapter explicates the Barry, Gordon & King Teaching/Learning Nursing Framework, which is a broad guide to study and analyze nursing situations that focuses on the caring between the nurse and one nursed. Through the study of nursing situations, students uncover the knowledge, skills, and practices most relevant to nursing.

The Barry, Gordon & King Teaching/Learning Nursing Framework is based on the foundational work of Boykin and Schoenhofer (2001); Florida Atlantic University, Christine E. Lynn College of Nursing's philosophy of nursing (2012); and Parker and Smith (2010). Building on this foundation, the authors expanded the framework to include additional ways of knowing, focused questions related to caring between the nurse and one nursed, and an evaluation of outcomes. The framework incorporates methods of reflective journaling and aesthetic re-presentations to facilitate students' deeper understanding of nursing.

STUDY PROCESSES

The Barry, Gordon & King Teaching/Learning Nursing Framework will be employed throughout this book. Using theoretical and philosophical perspectives of caring and multiple ways of knowing (Carper, 1978; Kagen, Smith, Cowling, & Chinn, 2009; Munhall, 1993; White, 1995), nursing situations are examined for the knowledge embedded within them. Nursing expertise is developed through intention, experience, study, and reflection on nursing situations.

Nursing situations were selected to reflect a cross section of populations, health concerns, and practice settings. Essential concepts reflecting recommendations from national reports and nursing scholars are embedded in select nursing situations. A crosswalk matrix organized around the intersections of population, physiological system, health concern, practice setting, caring concept, and essential concept for the nursing situations can be found in the Appendix.

The following questions were developed by the authors (Barry, Gordon, & King, 2013) and tested in teaching/learning environments over many years of education and practice. These questions, although not exhaustive, form the basis of engagement in the study of nursing situations and paths to knowing caring in specific nursing situations. They are offered as a guide to uncover nursing knowledge embedded in nursing situations and to provoke thoughtful reflection on caring as the central concept in nursing.

What Was the "Caring Between" the Nurse and the One Nursed?

The authors assert that nursing is a discipline and professional practice grounded in caring. An essential component of teaching/learning from nursing situations is the identification and explication of the caring between the nurse and one nursed. Using the caring components described by caring scholars (Mayeroff, 1971; Roach, 1987/2002), students are asked to describe expressions of caring and the essence of caring in nursing situations. Roach's essential attributes of caring—the Six Cs—provide a framework to teach and learn caring in nursing. Compassion is an intentional attempt to understand the other person's experience, pain and suffering, and happiness and joy that fosters the relationship between the nurse and one nursed. Competence is the knowing of the person, the judgment to respond appropriately, and the skill to care competently. As Roach (1987/2002) states, "While competence without compassion can be brutal and inhumane, compassion without competence may be no more than a meaningless, if not harmful, intrusion into the life of a person or persons needing help" (p. 54). Confidence is the nurse's ability to gain the trust of the other and trust in self. The development of a trusting relationship can enhance confidence in one another. Conscience is the moral component of nursing—doing what is right, knowing what is wrong, and taking action when needed. According to Roach (1987/2002), "conscience is the medium through which moral obligation is personalized" (p. 58). Commitment is fundamental to nursing; this is nursing's pledge to society and to the profession to care for others. Comportment is the nurse's demonstration of respect to self and the profession. Through comportment, the nurse can instill confidence, enhance the nurse–patient relationship, and honor the nursing profession.

Questions related to Roach's Six Cs might include:

- Was a call for compassion heard? How did you respond?
- How did you exhibit commitment to your patient?
- How did you demonstrate competence?
- How was your care guided by your conscience?

Mayeroff's (1971) philosophy of caring and caring ingredients is also used as a framework to understand caring. Caring is described as helping the other grow in his or her own time. Mayeroff asserts that this requires understanding the other not as a detached specimen, but as if you were in his or her world (pp. 53–54). The caring ingredients flow from this perspective and support the understanding of and attention to the other. The concepts of honesty, trust, knowing, alternating rhythms, patience, humility, hope, and courage translate easily to nursing and are useful in describing the essence of caring in a nursing situation. Honesty with self and the other is an essential ingredient in developing and maintaining a trusting relationship. Patience inspires the understanding that the other will grow and flourish in his or her own time and in his or her own way (p. 23). Understanding the alternating rhythms of relationships can facilitate a motion of being close and stepping away as the relationship ebbs and flows. Offering hope is an essential ingredient in nursing. Hope is a moment alive with possibilities that encourages spiritedness in the present time. Humility opens the door for the nurse to come to know and understand the hopes and dreams of the other.

Questions to facilitate understanding of caring may include:

- What happened between you and the one nursed?
- Which caring ingredient(s) guide your nursing practice?
- Is humility guiding my openness to know the one nursed?
- What was learned from the one nursed?

Using the Ways of Knowing, How Can We Come to Understand the Call(s) for Nursing?

Ways of knowing—personal, empirical, ethical, sociopolitical, spiritual, unknowing, emancipatory, and aesthetic—are used to understand the call for nursing in a given nursing situation (Carper, 1978; Kagen, Smith, Cowling, & Chinn, 2009; Munhall, 1993; White, 1995).

Personal knowing is a process of coming to understand self through self-reflection. Owning a sense of self-awareness assists in the development of personal knowing. Therapeutic use of self is often conceptualized as personal knowing in which the nurse and person strive to develop an authentic relationship of understanding and caring. Questions that reflect personal knowing may include:

- How do I understand myself as a caring person?
- Who is the one nursed as a caring person?
- What do I know from other similar situations that relate to this situation?
- What is the meaning of this situation to me?

Empirical knowing is a process of identifying, synthesizing, and applying the scientific evidence embedded in the nursing situation. This knowledge is systematically organized and based on laws and scientific theories that describe, explain, predict, and are verifiable. Human science provides valuable knowledge of the meaning of health experiences for the one nursed. Questions that reflect empirical knowing may include:

- What factual knowledge, laboratory results, medical reports, prescribed medications, and/or disease processes are evident?
- What research findings and evidence exists for best practice?
- What safety issues can be identified?
- What theory is useful to guide practice?

Ethical knowing is a process of understanding "right actions" in nursing situations, which are grounded in personal beliefs and professional values. Ethical knowing guides all intentional actions by the nurse. Questions that involve ethical knowing are:

- What components of the professional code of ethics are relevant?
- What should be done?
- Am I honest and truthful?
- Am I keeping the patient information confidential?
- Am I nonjudgmental?

Sociopolitical knowing is a process of understanding the context of a person's life and cultural influences. Questions to assist in understanding the sociopolitical knowing may include:

- What do I know about the individual's friends, family, partner(s), work, school, social life?
- What are the person's cultural beliefs?
- What do you know about the person's access to health care, safe housing, and leisure activities?
- What local, state, and federal policies and laws are impacting the well-being of the one nursed?

Spiritual knowing is a process of coming to understand the person's spiritual and religious beliefs, sense of belongingness, ritual practices, and inner sources of hope. Questions that reflect spiritual knowing may include:

- What are the person's and family's religious and/or spiritual beliefs and practices?
- What rituals are important to the person and family?
- How can hope be supported?

Unknowing is a process of suspending knowing to take in the fullness of the experience of the other. "Unknowing is different from not knowing" (Munhall, 2009, p. 164). It is listening with the third ear to what is not said and responding with an openness to know and understand the unique experience of the other. Questions that reflect unknowing are:

- How did I convey being authentically present?
- How can I be helpful to you or your family?
- What have I communicated nonverbally to the person and vice versa?
- How have I communicated being open to learn about the other? What did I learn about the person's thoughts and feelings?
- What matters most to you at this time?

Emancipatory knowing is a process of understanding barriers that create unfair and unjust social conditions that motivates action to improve people's lives (Chinn & Kramer, 2011, p. 248). Questions to assist in understanding emancipatory knowing may include:

- What barriers create unfair and unjust social conditions?
- What does it mean to be excluded from health care or medical decisions about oneself?
- What is the experience of nursing interactions that are disrespectful or lack compassion?
- What advocacy measures are needed to humanize and transform health care?

Aesthetic knowing is a process of artfully weaving together all ways of knowing in unity and fullness to create a meaningful caring moment in the nursing situation. Questions to assist in understanding aesthetic knowing are:

- How did all my knowing come together in this moment?
- What is the beauty of this situation?
- How can I transcend this moment to create possibilities?
- How have the arts influenced my practice?
- How can I represent this nursing situation in art form?

What Are the Calls for Nursing?

A call for nursing is a "call for acknowledgement and affirmation of the person" (Boykin & Schoenhofer, 1993, p. 24). Identification of the calls for nursing arises from the nurse's intentional engagement with the one nursed coupled with the nurse's broad knowledge base that heightens understanding in particular situations. The unique call for nursing reflects what is important to the one nursed at that moment in time. Touhy and Boykin (2008) recognize "the challenge for nursing is not to discover what is missing, weakened, or needed in another but to come to know the other as caring person and to nurture the person in situation specific, creative ways" (p. 12). Questions that help identify the call(s) are:

- What matters most to you at this time?
- How can I be helpful to you?
- How do I hear the unspoken calls for nursing?
- What do I know about this person that helps me identify calls for nursing?

What Are the Responses to the Calls for Nursing Present in the Situation?

The nurse's response to a call for nursing is a unique expression of caring. The creation of a response begins with reflection on knowing what it is to be human, what it means to live caring, and ways to nurture caring in each situation. The thoughtful intention and general knowledge the nurse brings to the situation is transformed into a response that reflects understanding and meaning of the uniqueness of the nursing situation. The nursing response grounded in caring acknowledges and affirms the other's wholeness and hopes and dreams for well-being. Questions assisting in the development of a response include:

- How did the response reflect the call for nursing?
- How did the ways of knowing inform the response(s) to the call?
- What other responses are possible?

What Was the Outcome of the Response?

Outcomes are changes that occur in response to nursing care as defined within a selected theoretical perspective. For example, using the philosophical lens of Florida Atlantic University's College of Nursing (2012), the intended outcome is nurturing the wholeness and well-being of the one nursed. Using the lens of Kolcaba's (2010) Comfort Theory, the outcome is enhanced comfort for the person. The outcome using Leininger's Theory of Cultural Care Diversity and Universality (Leininger & McFarland, 2010) would be culturally congruent care. Outcomes reflect the value of the response to the one nursed, the nurse, nursing colleagues, the profession, and significant others.

The following questions provide guidance to the evaluation of outcomes.

- What was the outcome of the nursing response?
- What was the influence of caring on the outcome?
- What evidence supports the effectiveness of the response?
- How does the outcome reflect the selected theoretical perspective?
- What was the rippling effect of the outcome?

How Did the Study of This Nursing Situation Enhance Your Knowledge of Nursing?

Nursing knowledge is embedded in nursing situations. Nursing expertise is developed through intention, experience, study, and reflection on nursing situations.

The following questions guide an evaluative process of teaching/ learning nursing from the context of nursing situations.

- What did I learn about myself?
- What did I learn about caring science?
- What did I learn about nursing science?
- What did I learn about interprofessional collaboration?
- What new possibilities can I create from this experience?

SUGGESTED LEARNING ACTIVITIES AND RESOURCES

Reflective Journaling

The goal of reflective journaling is to gain a greater understanding of self as a caring person and as a nurse. Reflective journaling has been described by Johns (2000) as a "place to listen and pay attention to one's own heartbeat of experience" (p. 45). Reflection is an inner dialogue with oneself to gain insights, to relate the ideal practice to the reality of practice, and to think through the nursing situation. The following guidelines are recommended to enter the world of reflective journaling.

Guidelines: The knowledge of nursing evolves through reflection, readings, and experience. Find a quiet place to reflect upon your nursing situation, and relive the sights, sounds, thoughts, and experiences while becoming reacquainted with the persons in the situation. Describe what happened between you and the one nursed.

The following questions focus on knowing the one nursed.

- Who is this person as a caring person?
- How does this person live caring day to day?
- What are this person's hopes and dreams?

- What are the calls for nursing?
- What have you learned from the different ways of knowing that enhanced your understanding of the call(s)?
- What are the possibilities of nursing responses?
- What is it like for me as person and a student to be in this clinical experience?
- How has reflection on the nursing situation enhanced my knowledge of nursing, caring, and nurturing of the other?
- What might I do differently next time?

Boxes 3.1 and 3.2 display excerpts from students' journals expressing growing understanding of nursing.

BOX 3.1   Reflective Journal: Excerpt From "Digging In"

Christie Bailey, MS, RN, AHN-BC

Now I am writing my journal and am up to 600 words. I am not nearly done with it.

The journal is going to be very long but, honestly, at this point, I am writing it for myself. It is causing me to go back to many sources of literature and ideas that I have had swirling in my head, and giving me a forum to synthesize all of it and...gel all of it together, I guess.

I think this is where all of my reading and learning is beginning to come together, here near the end of my PhD coursework, where I now have the beginnings of this rich foundation of knowledge.

Kind of reminds me of compost, actually. I've been laying down layers of knowledge, class after class, layer after layer, and letting it sit...and stirring it...and now I have this rich material to dip into!

BOX 3.2   Reflective Journal: From "Older Adult"

Rosemary Schiel, BSN, RN, CCM, CPHM

By coming to know this person as hopeful, loving, alert, and intellectually alive there are dreams of hers yet to be lived. This woman states, "I still am." She soars above the earth in her mind, which tells me that she still dreams and hopes to go, be, and do. Yet her joints hurt; her legs are thin, tired, and weak; and there is this call from her to nurture her wholeness.

My personal ways of knowing allows me to feel her aching and tired joints. My daughter has rheumatoid arthritis, so I know the pain and suffering of aching joints. Empirical knowing of human growth and development teaches me that the late stage of life is a stage of reflection. Ethical ways of knowing helps me to focus on the fact this person is no less of a person because they are old. Everyone will grow old if they live long enough. Society should look at the old as gifts, their pains are real and their care and concerns are important. We need to consider persons as people who are individuals with hopes and dreams of becoming. Aesthetic ways of knowing helps me to visualize who this person is with her beautiful spirit as she soars above the earth.

AESTHETIC RE-PRESENTATIONS

Aesthetic re-presentations are used to transform the nursing situation from words to an art form. Students are asked to reflect upon the meaning of their nursing situation and develop an aesthetic project that represents the essence of caring—the "in between" moment. Students discover their creative self to express the essence of caring in the nursing situation through reflection. Examples of aesthetic expressions include poetry, dance, music, drawings, plays, and art work. Directions to the student are kept to a minimum to allow the student to explore his or her own understanding of the essence of caring in the nursing situation.

Examples of Aesthetic Re-presentations

Art

Nurses are frequently called to create harmony within and amidst chaos. On September 11, 2001, the United States experienced an unprecedented attack on humanity. As part of a reflective assignment, nursing students were asked to create an aesthetic project representing their thoughts and feelings on this day.

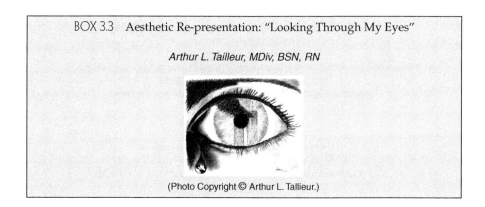

BOX 3.3   Aesthetic Re-presentation: "Looking Through My Eyes"

Arthur L. Tailleur, MDiv, BSN, RN

(Photo Copyright © Arthur L. Tallieur.)

Poetry

I can remember one time sharing a nursing situation with the class. It was about a person who was experiencing chronic cardiac distress, but he was really struggling with a nursing interaction. I was in the room with the person when another nurse came in to check his vital signs. As she approached him to listen to his heart, she said, off the cuff, "Do you have a heart?" His eyes filled with tears. I don't think the nurse saw his tears; she just left the room.

After the nurse left, we talked for a long time about what that meant to him, so I've used that story with students because it helps them understand all the different ways of knowing a person and engaging in a thoughtful process of being in that situation. Some said they would do the same because that is what they see modeled by other nurses.

Had the nurse entered from a thoughtful presence, she would not make light of the situation. It is easy to fall into that mindset when tasks become commonplace.

The call from the patient was to know him and what he was experiencing and to inspire hope. The nurse can never assume vital signs are just a reading. I don't think the nurse saw the tears. The doing is not what holds an extraordinary meaning to a person.

You can't plan for a nursing situation; they are spontaneous and begin by a reflecting question. It calls for each faculty and student to be in the nursing situation to appreciate the difference.

BOX 3.4   Aesthetic Re-presentation: The Poem, "The Need to Know"

Anne Boykin, PhD, RN

As you speak, I feel the pain of your tears
I watch as your nurse comes to listen to your heart and say,
"It's so faint. Is it there?"
You respond with tears—
"Please don't say that" as you frighteningly recall the doctor's words regarding
the severity of your cardiac condition
How your eyes beg for those who enter your room to know
Who you are
Your hopes and dreams
Your struggles and fears
Can't they know your heart is breaking?
Can they not hear your pleas?
I hold your hand and feel the common flow of our love, our energy
I know you as
Caring Person
Loving Person
Special Uncle
You know me as
Caring Person
Nurse
Special Niece
I am with you to share your journey

SUMMARY

This chapter describes the Barry, Gordon & King Teaching/Learning Nursing Framework and its usefulness in the study of nursing from nursing situations. An overview of the caring concepts of Mayeroff (1971) and Roach (2002) and ways of knowing (Carper, 1978; Kagen, Smith, Cowling, & Chinn, 2009; Munhall, 1993; White, 1995) are presented, along with reflective questions. Two learning activities, journaling, and aesthetic re-presentations are described and exemplars are included. A crosswalk matrix of essential concepts is described and found in the Appendix.

REFERENCES

Barry, C. D., Gordon, S. C., & King, B. (2013). Nursing situations: Teaching, learning and living caring in nursing [Abstract]. *International Journal for Human Caring, 17*(3), 50–51.

Boykin, A., & Schoenhofer, S. (1993). *Nursing as caring: A model for transforming practice*. New York, NY: National League for Nursing Press.

Boykin, A., & Schoenhofer, S. (2001). *Nursing as caring: A model for transforming practice*. Boston, MA: Jones & Bartlett Publishers.

Carper, B. (1978). Fundamental patterns of knowing. *Advances in Nursing Science, 1*(1), 13–24.

Chinn, P., & Kramer, M. (2011). *Integrated theory and knowledge development in nursing*. St. Louis, MO: Mosby/Elservier.

Florida Atlantic University, Christine E. Lynn College of Nursing. (2012). *Philosophy*. Retrieved from http://nursing.fau.edu/index.php?main=1&nav=635

Johns, C. (2000). *Becoming a reflective practitioner*. Oxford, UK: Blackwell Science Ltd.

Kagen, P. N., Smith, M. C., Cowling, R., & Chinn, P. (2009). A nursing manifesto: An emancipatory call for nursing knowledge development, conscience, and practice. *Nursing Philosophy, 11*(1), 67–84.

Kolcaba, K. (2010). Katherine Kolcaba's comfort theory. In M. Parker & M. Smith (Eds.), *Nursing theory and nursing practice* (3rd ed., pp. 389–401). Philadelphia, PA: F.A. Davis.

Leininger, M., & McFarland, M. R. (2010). The theory of culture care diversity and universality. In M. Parker & M. Smith (Eds.), *Nursing theory and nursing practice* (3rd ed., pp. 317–336). Philadelphia, PA: F.A. Davis.

Mayeroff, M. (1971). *On caring*. New York, NY: HarperCollins.

Munhall, P. (1993). Unknowing: Toward another pattern of knowing. *Nursing Outlook, 41*, 125–128.

Munhall, P. L. (2009). Unknowing: Towards the understanding of multiple realities and manifold perceptions. In R. Locsin & M. Purnell (Eds.), *A contemporary nursing process: The (un)bearable weight of knowing in nursing* (pp. 153–173). New York, NY: Springer.

Parker, M., & Smith, M. (Eds.). (2010). *Nursing theories & nursing practice* (3rd ed.). Philadelphia, PA: F.A. Davis.

Roach, M. S. (1987/2002). *Caring, the human mode of being: A blueprint for the health professions (2nd rev. ed)*. Ottawa, Canada: The Canadian Hospital Association Press.

Roach, M. S. (2002). *The human act of caring: A blueprint for the health professions*. Ottawa, Canada: The Canadian Hospital Association Press.

Touhy, T., & Boykin, A. (2008). Caring as the central domain in nursing. *International Journal for Human Caring, 12*(2), 9–15.

White, J. (1995). Patterns of knowing: Review, critique, and update. *Advances in Nursing Science, 17*(4), 73–86.

Understanding the Framework for Studying Nursing Situations From Selected Nursing Theoretical Perspectives

Nursing theoretical frameworks provide theory-based approaches to the study of nursing. Chapter 4 recognizes the variety of nursing theoretical perspectives used in teaching/learning. Guiding questions to facilitate the study of nursing through the use of nursing situations from the Barry, Gordon & King Teaching/Learning Nursing Framework and selected theoretical perspectives are provided.

BARRY, GORDON & KING TEACHING/LEARNING NURSING FRAMEWORK

The Barry, Gordon & King Teaching/Learning Nursing Framework is based on the foundational work of Boykin and Schoenhofer (2001), Florida Atlantic University College of Nursing's philosophy of nursing (FAU, CON, 2012), and Parker and Smith (2010). The guiding questions of the framework for studying nursing through nursing situations presented in Chapter 3 were adapted, in part, from Parker and Smith's approach to thinking about nursing theory. Table 4.1 provides a visual display of selected reflective questions

TABLE 4.1 Questions Regarding Thinking About a Nursing Theory

What is the visual model of the theory?
What is the focus of nursing?
What are the assumptions and beliefs of the theory?
What is the nurse doing when practicing from this theory/model?
What are the sources for studying and learning nursing?
What is created in and through nursing that makes outcomes possible?
What is the outcome(s) of nursing?

Source: Parker and Smith (2010).

developed by Parker and Smith as a beginning tool to study nursing situations from a theoretical perspective.

Parker and Smith's approach bases thinking about a nursing theory within the theory's usefulness as a means to guide the practice of nursing. Through a series of thoughtful questions, they invite the reader to visualize the model against the backdrop of his or her practice; this allows the reader to imagine what the nurse is focusing on when thinking about nursing from the perspective of a specific model, what the nurse is doing when practicing from the model, what the nurse is uniquely creating through theory-based practice, and the possible nursing outcomes derived from practicing nursing from the perspective of the model being studied.

Thinking about nursing is facilitated through use of narrative pedagogy as described by Diekelmann (1990). Nursing situations, as lived experiences of caring between in nursing practice, provide an opportunity for teachers and students to come together for the purpose of engaging in a focused conversation about the study of nursing and nursing practice. Questions designed to guide learners to think about nursing from the perspective of a selected nursing theory combined with narratives from nursing practice create opportunities for deep conversations. This approach to the study of nursing moves students away from focusing on finding the right answer and opens a shared exploration of the possibilities that live within each unique nursing situation. See Table 4.2 for examples of guiding questions reflecting the Barry, Gordon & King Teaching/Learning Nursing Framework.

FACILITATING THE STUDY OF NURSING SITUATIONS USING SELECTED THEORETICAL PERSPECTIVES

Chapters 5 through 20 present exemplars of the study of nursing through nursing situations across the practice spectrum using guiding questions developed from the Teaching/Learning Nursing Framework approach developed by Barry, Gordon, and King. However, the heuristic approach of

TABLE 4.2   Guiding Questions: Teaching/Learning Nursing Framework

What is the focus of nursing?

Nurturing the wholeness of others and environment in caring (FAU, CON, 2012).

What is the call for nursing?

Identification of the calls for nursing arises from the intentional full engagement of the nurse with the one nursed and from the nurse's ability to draw on a broad knowledge base in order to understand particular situations (Touhy & Boykin, 2008).

What ways of knowing are used to understand the call for nursing?

- Personal knowing: How do I understand and know myself as a caring person? Who is the person as a caring person? What is the meaning of this situation to me? What do I know from other situations?
- Empirical knowing: What is the factual knowledge of this situation? What are the laboratory results, medications, and disease processes? What evidence exists for best practice? What caring science is present in this situation?
- Ethical knowing: What components of the ethical codes for nurses are present in this situation? What are nursing's values? What should be done? Am I honest and truthful? Am I keeping the patient information confidential? Am I nonjudgmental?
- Sociopolitical knowing: What is the context of the person's life—friends, family, partner, work, spirituality? What are the person's responsibilities? What are the person's cultural beliefs? Does the person have access to health care, safe housing, and leisure activities? How can I help support the other? What health policy factors are evident?
- Unknowing: Tell me how it feels to be you? What matters most to you at this time? Unknowing is different from not knowing. Unknowing is the art of suspending knowing to take in the fullness of the experience of the other. It is listening with the *third ear* to what is not said and responding with an openness to know and understand the unique experience of the other.
- Emancipatory knowing: What does it mean to be excluded from health care and medical decisions about oneself? What does it feel like to be known by the health concern, such as being called the diabetic or the fracture or the open heart in bed 3? What is it like to lack access to health care for self and family? What is it like to receive care that is not grounded in respect and compassion? What does it take to humanize and transform health care?
- Aesthetic knowing: All ways of knowing are gathered together in unity and fullness in the nursing situation, wholeness, caring, oneness, valuing the in-between, and beyond. What is the beauty of this situation? How have the arts influenced my practice? How can I support my patient's hopes and dreams? How can I transcend this moment to create possibilities? What metaphors might express the meaning of this situation?

What is the nursing response to the call?

The nurse brings knowing what it is to be human, what is means to live caring, and how to nurture wholeness and well-being in each situation. The general knowledge the nurse brings to the situation is transformed to provide meaning and understanding of the uniqueness of the situation. To acknowledge, affirm, and sustain the other's hopes and dreams for well-being.

- How did each way of knowing inform the nursing response?

(continued)

TABLE 4.2   Guiding Questions: Teaching/Learning Nursing
Framework (*continued*)

What is the outcome of the response in relation to the call?
■ What is the value of the response to the one nursed, the nurse, nursing colleagues, the profession, and significant others? ■ How did each way of knowing inform an understanding of the outcome?

Source: King, Barry, & Gordon (2014).

teaching/learning nursing from nursing situations can be adapted to any nursing theoretical framework. This chapter presents guiding questions for selected nursing theoretical perspectives that are commonly utilized in schools of nursing, practice settings, and research. A brief description of selected grand and midrange theories is presented. Readers are encouraged to review the relevant literature to support a full understanding of each theoretical perspective.

The guiding questions are not intended to be exhaustive. They are designed to provide a starting place for a theoretical approach to the study of nursing situations. When used to study nursing through a unique nursing situation, the guiding questions presented in this chapter and subsequent teacher–student conversations can be adapted to reflect the uniqueness of nursing situations, personal experiences of the readers, and/or planned learning objectives. They also serve as a roadmap to develop guiding questions for additional theoretical frameworks with the intent of teaching/learning nursing from nursing situations.

SELECTED GRAND THEORIES

Grand theories, also known as conceptual models, are highly abstract and represent a compilation of broad concepts and statements of relationship between concepts. In nursing, the intent of grand theories is to describe the whole of the discipline across practice settings and serve as a practice blueprint describing what the nurse is thinking about and doing when practicing. Examples of grand theory include: Theory of Caring (Watson, 2008), Nursing as Caring (Boykin & Schoenhofer, 2001), Theory of Culture Care Diversity and Universality (Leininger, 2002), and the Self-Care Deficit Nursing Theory (Orem, 1991). Following a brief description of each theory, guiding questions translated from the Barry, Gordon & King Teaching/Learning Nursing Framework for the study of nursing through nursing situations is presented. The guiding questions can be used to study the nursing situations presented in Chapters 5 through 20.

WATSON'S THEORY OF HUMAN CARING

The major conceptual elements of Watson's 1985 Theory of Human Caring include 10 carative factors, caring moments, caring–healing modalities, and transpersonal caring relationships (Watson & Woodward, 2010, p. 353). Recently, Watson has reframed carative factors as "caritas processes" and "clinical caritas." Caritas connotes love and "allows love and caring to come together to form deep transpersonal caring" (p. 353). Caring moments are created through the use of caring–healing modalities.

For Watson, transpersonal caring relationships move beyond ego self to connect with spiritual concerns that allow the nurse to access healing possibilities and potentials (p. 356). It is her belief that the one caring and the one being cared for are interconnected in a transpersonal caring relationship and "the whole caring–healing consciousness is contained within a single caring–healing moment" (p. 357). From this perspective, the focus of nursing is the transpersonal caring relationship between the nurse and the ones being cared for that creates harmony, wholeness, and unity of being in caring moments. See Table 4.3 for examples of guiding questions formatted from the Barry, Gordon & King Teaching/Learning Nursing Framework to reflect Watson's Theory of Human Caring.

BOYKIN AND SCHOENHOFER'S THEORY OF NURSING AS CARING

The main assumption of the Theory of Nursing as Caring (Boykin & Schoenhofer, 1993) is drawn from Roach's early thesis, "caring is the human mode of being" (1987/2002, p. 28). The formative ideas of call and response, nursing response, and personhood form the structural basis for the theory. In addition, Mayeroff's (1971) caring ingredients were incorporated to provide the practical language of caring in nursing situations. Caring is defined as an "altruistic, active expression of love and is the intentional and embodied recognition of value and connectedness" (Boykin, Schoenhofer, & Linden, 2010, p. 372). However, the theorists caution the full meaning of caring cannot be expressed in a conceptual definition.

The theorists defined the term *nursing situation* as "a shared lived experience in which the caring between nurse and nursed enhances personhood" (Boykin, Schoenhofer, & Linden, 2010, p. 372). They assert it is in the *in-between* that caring is lived between the nurse and the one nursed. Therefore, "the practical knowledge of nursing lives within the context of person-to-person caring" (2010, p. 372). "From the perspective of the Theory of Nursing as Caring, the focus of nursing is person as living and growing in caring" (Boykin, Schoenhofer, & Linden, 2010, p. 372). Nurses respond to unique calls for nursing that are heard from individuals. The theorists describe a call for nursing as "a call for acknowledgement and affirmation of the person living caring in specific ways in the immediate situation" (Boykin

TABLE 4.3   Guiding Questions: Theory of Human Caring

■ What is the focus of nursing?   The transpersonal caring relationship between the nurse and the ones being cared for that creates harmony, wholeness, and unity of being in caring moments.
■ How do I enter the life space of another to detect the other's condition of being?   How do I authentically connect with another with intention? How do I move beyond ego to embrace the spirit of another? What strategies assist me to be present to self and others?
■ What knowledge is needed to understand a caring science orientation to nursing?   Scientific: What caring science is present in this situation?   Aesthetic: How can I seek "authentic, caring connections and caring–healing relationships" (p. 356) in this situation? How can I transform or improve practice to reflect caring science? How can I transcend this moment to create moments?   Ethic: Is there congruence with my values and the practice setting necessary to transform or improve practice from the perspective of caring science? What is my view of being human?   Major factors studied from the perspective of the Theory of Human Caring include 10 clinical caritas processes and a transpersonal caring relationship.
■ How can I create a practice of loving kindness within the context of human science? How can I enable and sustain the subjective life world of self and other? How can I be open to others with sensitivity and compassion? What approaches are useful in developing authentic, caring relationships? How can I promote and accept expressions of positive and negative feelings? What problem-solving caring processes support the creative use of self? How do I present teaching/learning from within the other's frame of reference? What environmental factors in this nursing situation support a healing environment? What knowledge is needed to intentionally administer human care essentials? How do I attend to soul care in this nursing situation? How do I "center consciousness and intentionality on caring, healing, and wholeness, rather than on disease, illness, and pathology" (p. 357)?
■ What caring–healing modalities "potentiate harmony, wholeness, and unity of being" in this nursing situation? (p. 358)
■ Were the individual's "subjective inner healing processes" (p. 357) supported through a transpersonal caring relationship?   ■ How did the nurse focus intentionally on caring and creating harmony, wholeness, and unity of being in caring moments?

Source: Watson and Woodward (2010).

& Schoenhofer, 1993, p. 24). Nursing responses are expressions of nursing in which the nurse is intentionally present with another who is recognized as living and growing in caring. The value of nursing is expressed as arising in and evolving through the "caring between of the nursing situation" (Boykin, Schoenhofer, & Linden, 2010, p. 379). Therefore, the value of nursing cannot be measured as discrete predetermined outcomes. See Table 4.4 for examples of guiding questions formatted from the Barry, Gordon & King Teaching/Learning Nursing Framework to reflect Boykin and Schoenhofer's Theory of Nursing as Caring.

TABLE 4.4   Guiding Questions: Nursing as Caring

■ What is the focus of nursing? How is this person living and growing in caring? Was personhood of the nurse and the one nursed enhanced?
■ What is the call for nursing? How do I acknowledge and affirm persons living caring in specific ways in the immediate nursing situation? How can I nurture this person to grow in caring?
■ What ways of knowing are used to understand the call for nursing? Personal knowing: How do I understand and know myself as a caring person? How do I know this person as living and growing in caring? What is the meaning of this situation to me? What do I know from other situations? Empirical knowing: What is the factual knowledge of this situation? What are the lab results, medications, and disease processes? What evidence exists for best practice? What caring science is present in this situation? Ethical knowing: What components of the ethical codes for nurses are present in this situation? What are nursing's values? What should be done? Am I honest and truthful? Am I keeping the patient information confidential? Am I nonjudgmental? Sociopolitical knowing: What is the context of the person's life—friends, family, partner, work, and spirituality? What are the person's responsibilities? What are the person's cultural beliefs? Does the person have access to health care, safe housing, and leisure activities? How can I help support the other? What health policy factors are evident? Aesthetic knowing: All ways of knowing are gathered together in unity and fullness in the nursing situation, wholeness, caring, oneness, valuing the in between, and beyond. What is the beauty of this situation? How have the arts influenced my practice? How can I support my patient's hopes and dreams? How can I transcend this moment to create possibilities? What metaphors might express the meaning of this situation?
Nursing Response ■ As I intentionally entered into the nursing situation, was I authentically present with another? ■ Did I recognize the person as living and growing in caring?
Nursing Outcome What was experienced as "arising in and evolving through the 'caring between' of the nursing situation" (Boykin, Schoenhofer, & Linden, 2010, p. 379)? ■ Was personhood of the nurse and the one nursed enhanced?

Source: Boykin and Schoenhofer (2001).

OREM'S SELF-CARE DEFICIT NURSING THEORY

Orem's (2001) Self-Care Deficit Nursing Theory is an action theory that focuses on role specifications for nurses and patients. Within the context of the theory, Orem identifies two categories of people—those who need nursing and those who produce it.

Self-Care Deficit Nursing Theory is composed of three midrange theories: the Theory of Self-Care (detailed knowledge of universal, health deviation, and developmental self-care requisites), the Theory of Self-Care agency (detailed knowledge of characteristics that determine power available to act in one's own behalf to accomplish self-care), and the Theory of Nursing Systems (three levels of care systems based on intensity and extensity of modes of helping involved in nurse agency to act on another's behalf to accomplish self-care or to support self-care agency).

Major concepts in the Self-Care Deficit Nursing Theory include four patient-related concepts (self-care/dependent care, self-care agency/dependent-care agency, therapeutic self-care demand, and self-care deficit/dependent-care deficit) and two nurse-related concepts (nursing agency and nursing system). The basic conditioning factors concept is a peripheral concept relating to both the patient and the nurse.

The concepts of self-care, agency, therapeutic self-care demand, self-care deficit, and nursing systems are integral to understanding the theory. Self-care is "the practice of activities that individuals initiate and perform on their own behalf in maintaining life, health, and well-being" (p. 43). Orem (2001) defines agent as the "person who engages in a course of action or has the power to do so" (p. 514). Agent and agency apply to both the patient and the nurse. Therapeutic self-care demand refers to all actions a patient should perform to meet self-care needs. A self-care deficit occurs when an individual is unable to meet his or her therapeutic self-care demand. Nursing is needed whenever a self-care deficit occurs. As defined by Orem, nursing systems are action systems that represent actions taken by nurses for or with a self-care agent to promote life, health, and well-being. The goal of nurse agency is "to know and meet a patient's therapeutic self-care demands and to protect and to regulate the exercise and development of a patient's self-care agency" (p. 290). See Table 4.5 for examples of guiding questions formatted from the Barry, Gordon & King Teaching/Learning Nursing Framework to reflect Orem's Self-Care Deficit Nursing Theory.

ROY'S ADAPTATION MODEL

Roy's Adaptation Model (Roy, 2009) is based, in part, on the theoretical assumptions of von Bertalanffy's (1968) General Systems Theory, Helson's (1964) Adaptation-Level Theory, and Young's (1986) beliefs about the unity and meaningfulness of the universe. Major concepts of the theory include

TABLE 4.5   Guiding Questions: Self-Care Deficit Nursing Theory

What is the proper object and focus of nursing?

Persons experiencing self-care deficits and receiving nursing care are the proper objects of nursing. The object is "to know and meet patients' therapeutic self-care demands and to protect and regulate the exercise of patients' self-care agency" (Orem, 2001, p. 290).

What self-care deficits require nursing?

Identification of self-care deficits that arise from the nurse's evaluation of the relationship between an individual's self-care agency and therapeutic self-care demands. When a patient's self-care agency is not adequate to meet self-care demands for action to achieve self-care requisites or anticipated self-care requisites, a self-care deficit exists and legitimate nursing is required (Hartweg & Fleck, 2010).

What knowledge is used to understand self-care deficits and nursing systems?

Major elements studied from the perspective of the Self-Care Deficit Nursing Theory are the theory of self-care (detailed knowledge of universal, health deviation, and developmental self-care requisites), the theory of self-care agency (detailed knowledge of characteristics that determine power available to act in one's own behalf to accomplish self-care), and the theory of nursing systems (three levels of care systems based on intensity and extensity of modes of helping involved in nurse agency to act in another's behalf to accomplish self-care or to support self-care agency; Orem, 2001).

- What is the therapeutic self-care demand for action in this situation? Review each of the universal requisites, in relation to the health concern.
- What is the individual's power to act in his or her own behalf in this situation to accomplish self-care, and what are the limitations on self-care action?
- What is the balance between therapeutic self-care demand for action and the power of self-care agency in this situation? Specify that balance as a statement of self-care deficit.

What nursing actions were taken to meet self-care deficits and anticipated self-care deficits?

The nurse designs nursing systems to address calculated self-care deficits and anticipated self-care deficits.

- How did the nurse enter into an interpersonal relationship with the patient in this situation?
- What guiding, supporting, and protecting actions were implemented to meet therapeutic self-care demands?
- What actions were completed for or with the patient (self-care agent) in this situation to promote life, health, and well-being?
- Who performed these actions in this situation?
- Who should have performed these actions?
- What control operations were used to appraise and evaluate the effectiveness of the nursing actions?
- What actions could have been used?
- What was the essence of nursing (caring) in this situation?

(*continued*)

TABLE 4.5 Guiding Questions: Self-Care Deficit Nursing Theory (*continued*)

Nursing Outcome What was the product of the nursing system? ■ To what extent were self-care deficits resolved? ■ What modifications in the original nursing system design were needed in order to achieve required care?

Source: Orem (2001).

people (individuals and groups) as adaptive systems, health, environment, and the goal of nursing. Roy focuses on people (individuals and groups) as holistic adaptive systems that act to maintain adaptation and promote person and environment transformations through the use of coping processes (Roy & Zhan, 2010). Coping processes (cognator–regulator and stabilizer–innovator) are focused on stability and change. Categories of coping activity are called adaptive modes. The adaptive modes include physiologic–physical, self-concept–group identity, role function, and interdependence.

Environment is defined as "all the conditions, circumstances, and influences surrounding and affecting the development and behavior of individuals and groups" (Roy & Zhan, 2010, p. 173). Internal and external environmental factors (focal, contextual, and residual stimuli) serve as input for the adaptive system. Internal and external stimuli may lead to compromised adaptation by the system (individuals or group).

Health is defined by Roy as "the reflection of personal and environmental interactions that are adaptive" (Roy & Zhan, 2010, pp. 173–174). The goal of nursing is the "promotion of adaptation for individuals and groups in each of the four adaptive modes, thus contributing to health, quality of life, and dying with dignity" (Roy & Zhan, 2010, p. 174). See Table 4.6 for examples of guiding questions formatted from the Barry, Gordon & King Teaching/Learning Nursing Framework to reflect Roy's Adaptation Model.

TABLE 4.6 Guiding Questions: The Roy Adaptation Model

■ What is the focus of nursing?
"The Roy Adaptation Model focuses on enhancing the basic life processes of the individual and group" (Roy & Zhan, 2010, p. 272).
■ What is the call for nursing?
"To promote the individual's coping and adaptation processing in the context of health and illness" (Roy & Zhan, 2010, p. 277).

(*continued*)

TABLE 4.6   Guiding Questions: The Roy Adaptation Model (*continued*)

What knowledge is used to understand individual or group coping and adaptation processing and self-consistency?

Major elements studied from the perspective of the Roy Adaptation Model include coping and adaptation processing and self-consistency. The relationship between the constructs cognator and regulator processes and affective adaptive responses is an essential assumption of the model.

- What cognator and regulator processes of the individual and innovator and stabilizer of the group promote adaptation?

Human adaptation occurs through cognitive processes:

- What input processes (arousal and attention, sensation and perception) promote adaptation?
- What central processes (coding, concept formation, memory, language) promote adaptation?
- What output processes (planning and motor responses) promote adaptation?
- What is the person's or group's adaptive ability to maintain self-consistency and system balance?
- What ineffective behaviors are demonstrated by the individual or group?

What is the adequacy of the patient's cognator and regulator processes and self-consistency?

- How can the nurse assist people or groups "in using cognitive abilities to handle internal and external environment effectively" (Roy & Zhan, 2010, p. 272)?
- What environmental stimuli could the nurse manipulate to enhance the basic life processes of the individual or group and promote self-consistency?

To what extent has the individual or group achieved system balance?

- What modifications in the original nursing system design are needed to assist the individual or group achieve system balance?

Source: Roy (2009).

LEININGER'S THEORY OF CULTURE CARE DIVERSITY AND UNIVERSALITY

Leininger (1991) developed the Theory of Culture Care Diversity and Universality to provide nurses with the knowledge base needed to develop transcultural nursing practices necessary in providing culturally sensitive, meaningful care. Leininger believed nurses needed to be prepared to care for people of many different cultures worldwide in response to global migrations of people following World War II. Factors influencing the development of her theory included observations of nurse stressors related to caring for culturally diverse populations, consumer fears associated with unfamiliar technologies and treatments, consumer frustration with nurses' misunderstanding of cultural beliefs and practices, misdiagnoses and mistreatment based on cultural misunderstandings, intercultural conflict and pain, limited diversity of health personnel, and increased number of nurses working in foreign countries (Leininger & McFarland, 2010).

Commonalities that are found within cultures are an important tenet of the Theory of Culture Care Diversity and Universality. Nurses intentionally look for the care values and patterns embedded within cultures in order to provide therapeutic outcomes. Leininger believed discovering which elements of care were universal and which were varied by culture would revolutionize nursing care.

The influence of worldview and social structure factors on health care outcomes is another major tenet of the Theory of Culture Care Diversity and Universality. This tenet provides a holistic view of understanding people within a historical context. It provides insight into providing culturally sensitive care through the development of culturally congruent, holistic, culture nursing knowledge.

Another major tenet of the theory is recognition of the influence of professional and generic or "folk" care practices on the health and well-being of individuals, family groups, or communities. Leininger introduced the importance of nurses identifying the similarities and differences in the care practices in order to recognize harmful care practices or significant gaps in health care.

Culture care preservation or maintenance, accommodation or negotiation, and restructuring or repatterning were identified by Leininger as nursing modalities focused on attaining or maintaining culturally congruent care. The culture care modalities and tenets of the Theory of Culture Care Diversity and Universality are depicted in Leininger's Sunrise Model (Leininger, 1991, p. 325). The model presents a guide to understanding the complex factors that influence cultural health care assessment of individuals, family groups, or communities and the provision of culturally congruent care. See Table 4.7 for examples of guiding questions formatted from the Barry, Gordon & King Teaching/Learning Nursing Framework to reflect Leininger's Theory of Culture Care Diversity and Universality.

TABLE 4.7 Guiding Questions: The Theory of Culture Care Diversity and Universality

■ What is the focus of nursing?
To provide culture-specific congruent and competent care to assist or improve one's health and well-being or to face illness, disability, or death.
■ What is the call for transcultural nursing?
To provide care that is beneficial, satisfying, and meaningful.

(continued)

TABLE 4.7   Guiding Questions: The Theory of Culture Care Diversity
and Universality (*continued*)

What knowledge is needed to understand transcultural nursing?

■ Culture care diversity: What "differences in meanings, patterns, values, lifeways, or symbols of care within or between cultures that demonstrate assistive, supportive, or enabling human care expressions" are present in this nursing situation (Leininger, 1991, p. 47)?
■ Culture care universality: What are the "common or dominant uniform care meanings, patterns, values, lifeways, or symbols of care" present in this situation that "reflect assistive, supportive, or enabling ways to assist people" (Leininger, 1991, p. 47)?
■ Culture care preservation: What "assistive, supportive, facilitative, and enabling professional care actions" are needed to "assist the client to preserve relevant care values" (Leininger, 1991, p. 48)? How can the nurse determine relevant care values and evaluate culture care preservation?
■ Culturalogical health assessment: What knowledge is needed to guide a culturalogical health care assessment? What ideas or experiences about care are relevant to the client? What culture care phenomena are discovered? What worldview is embraced by the client? How can I hold my worldview in abeyance?
■ Generic folk and lay care: What generic folk and lay care knowledge or skills guide client decisions and actions? How can generic folk and lay care practices be incorporated into the client's plan of care?

Other knowledge needed:

■ Kinship and social: What cultural beliefs, values, and recurrent lifeways arise from transgenerational linkages? How do social interactions influence cultural beliefs, values, and recurrent lifeways?
■ Economic: What economic factors influence the client's actions, decisions, and behaviors that impact health and well-being? What resources are available to assist the client?
■ Political and legal: What political and legal factors influence the client's actions, decisions, and behaviors that have the potential to impact health and well-being?
■ Environment: What geographic environmental factors influence the client's actions, decisions, and behaviors that have the potential to impact health and well-being? What ecological environmental factors influence the client's actions, decisions, and behaviors that have the potential to impact health and well-being?
■ Religious and philosophical: What spiritual and philosophical factors influence health and well-being?
■ Technological factors: What technological factors influence health and well-being (transportation, computer, communication, cell phones)?
■ Education: What formal and informal modes of learning influence the client's actions, decisions, and behaviors? How does the client acquire knowledge about ideas and subjects?

What care expressions facilitate culturally meaningful and therapeutic health and healing outcomes?

The nurse brings culturally based care knowledge and action modes in beneficial and meaningful ways to assist or improve the client's health and well-being and/or to face illness and death.

■ What health and healing actions were developed with the client?
■ How did the nurse and client work together to create meaningful action modes?

(*continued*)

TABLE 4.7 Guiding Questions: The Theory of Culture Care Diversity and Universality (*continued*)

What is the outcome of transcultural nursing care?
■ How did Leininger's model inform the practice of nursing? Did the client experience culture-specific congruent and competent care? ■ Did the client experience improved health and well-being or was he or she assisted to face illness, disability, or death in the context of his or her cultural expressions? ■ What transcultural knowledge and practices supported the outcomes?

Source: Leininger (1991).

MIDRANGE THEORIES

Unlike grand theories, theories of the middle range are broad enough to be useful in complex situations and narrow enough to guide empirical testing more easily. Midrange theories have a narrower scope of phenomena and are less abstract. Smith and Liehr (2008) suggest that because middle range theories have a narrower scope than grand theories, they may be more effective in increasing theory-based research and nursing practice intervention. Smith (2008) provides a framework for the evaluation of middle range theories. She offers criteria developed specifically for middle range theories related to substantive foundations (the fit of the theory with the focus of nursing), structural integrity (concept definitions and logical connections between concepts), and functional adequacy (application of the theory to nursing practice).

Comfort Theory (Kolcaba, 2010) and Theory of Uncertainty in Illness (Mishel, 1988) are examples of theories of the middle range. The guiding questions in the chapter tables have been reframed from the Barry, Gordon & King Teaching/Learning Nursing Framework for use in expanding the study of the nursing situations presented in Chapters 5 through 20 in this book.

KOLCABA'S COMFORT THEORY

Kolcaba (2010) defines comfort as a complex "outcome of intentional, patient/family-focused, quality care" (p. 390). Assumptions guiding Comfort Theory include the following: comfort is a basic human need, persons experience comfort holistically, self-comforting behaviors can be healthy or unhealthy, and enhanced comfort leads to increased productivity (p. 390).

Comfort can be understood and experienced in four contexts: physical, psychospiritual, sociocultural, and environmental. Kolcaba's taxonomy of comfort considers the contexts of comfort with the types of comfort that include relief, ease, and transcendence. Nurses can use this taxonomic structure to create patterns of comfort care for patients and family members. From the perspective of Comfort Theory, the outcome of comfort is "[t]he immediate relief of being strengthened when needs for relief, ease, and transcendence are addressed in four contexts of experience" (p. 390). See Table 4.8 for guiding questions formatted from the Barry, Gordon & King Teaching/ Learning Nursing Framework to reflect Kolcaba's Comfort Theory.

TABLE 4.8   Guiding Questions: Comfort Theory

What is the focus of nursing?
■ Enhancing patient comfort.
Comfort needs What are the physical and emotional comfort needs of the individual? ■ Comfort needs are met in the contexts of experience: physical, psychospiritual, social, and environmental.
Knowledge needed to enhance comfort What knowledge is needed to understand enhanced comfort? ■ How do I intentionally assess the physical, psychospiritual, social, and environmental health care needs of the patient/family? ■ What intervening variables impact comfort? Intervening factors such as prognosis, financial situation, and extent of social support do not change readily and are factors that nurses need to understand but often have little control over. ■ What patient and family internal or external health-seeking behaviors increase or decrease comfort? ■ What are the desired health-seeking behaviors to increase comfort? "Health-Seeking Behavior (HSBs) can be internal (healing, immune function, number of T cells, etc.), external (health related activities, functional outcomes, etc.), or a peaceful death" (Kolcaba, 2010, p. 393). ■ What best practices enhance comfort for individual patients and families? ■ How does the comfort level of patients and families impact institutional integrity? Institutional integrity is defined as the values, financial stability, and wholeness of health care organizations at local, regional, state, and national levels (Kolcaba, 2010). ■ How can institutional integrity be operationally defined? Possible measures of institutional integrity include: patient satisfaction, improved access, decreased morbidity rates, decreased hospitalizations and readmissions, improved health-related outcomes, efficiency of services and billing, positive cost-benefit ratios, and increased nurse satisfaction and retention rates. ■ What best institutional policies promote an environment supportive of enhanced patient and family comfort?

(continued)

TABLE 4.8 Guiding Questions: Comfort Theory (*continued*)

Nursing interventions What comforting interventions enhance comfort?   ■ Nurses intentionally assess the individual's needs for relief, ease, and transcendence (Kolcaba, 2010).
Nursing outcomes To what extent was comfort enhanced for individual patients and families?   ■ What modifications in nursing comfort interventions were needed to enhance comfort?   ■ How can I create patterns of comfort to meet the patient's or family members' needs for relief, ease, and transcendence?

Source: Kolcaba (2010).

MISHEL'S THEORY OF UNCERTAINTY

The Theory of Uncertainty in Illness was developed by Mishel in 1988 and reconceptualized in 1990. The reconceptualized Theory of Uncertainty in Illness "address[es] the process that occurs when a person lives with unremitting uncertainty found in chronic illness or in illness with a potential for recurrence" (Mishel & Clayton, 2008, p. 56). Mishel asserts there is a negative relationship between level of uncertainty and a person's ability to determine meaning regarding specific illness-events. The purpose of the theory is to explain the process through which persons "move from uncertainty appraised as danger to uncertainty appraised as an opportunity and resource ... for a new view of life" (p. 62). The theory is composed of themes related to antecedents of uncertainty, appraisal of uncertainty, and coping with uncertainty. The goal or "desired outcome of the reconceptualized Theory of Uncertainty in Illness is growth to a new value system" (p. 56). The following table reframes the guiding questions from the Barry, Gordon & King Teaching/Learning Nursing Framework to reflect Mishel's Theory of Uncertainty in Illness (Table 4.9).

Chapter 4 presents guiding questions supporting teaching/learning nursing from nursing situations from the perspective of the Barry, Gordon & King Teaching/Learning Nursing Framework and selected grand and midrange nursing theoretical perspectives commonly utilized in schools of nursing, practice settings, and guiding nursing research. The guiding questions in this chapter are intended to support the translation of nursing situations presented from the perspective of the teaching/learning framework (presented in Chapters 5 through 20) to selected, widely used theoretical perspectives. Learners are encouraged to refer to this chapter when reviewing the presented nursing situations and to develop additional questions that guide their understanding of nursing through the study of nursing situations.

TABLE 4.9   Guiding Questions: Theory of Uncertainty in Illness

■ What is the focus of nursing? Assisting patients to manage uncertainty in illness.
Nursing Interventions ■ What nursing interventions are effective in assisting patients to develop skills needed to manage uncertainty in illness? Nursing interventions effective in assisting patients to develop skills to manage uncertainty in illness focus on problem solving, cognitive reframing, patient–provider communication, and such. Knowledge needed to understand uncertainty ■ What knowledge is used to understand uncertainty in illness? ■ How do I understand the patient's level of uncertainty in illness and the impact of uncertainty on his or her illness experience?
What intervening variables impact uncertainty? ■ What intervening variables such as *stimuli frame* impact an individual's perceived uncertainty? What symptom patterns impact uncertainty? ■ Has a diagnosis been shared with the patient and family? ■ What symptoms are identified? ■ Can symptoms be attributed to a particular diagnosis? ■ How well is the patient managing existing symptoms? How does event congruence impact uncertainty? ■ How predictable are the symptoms? ■ What is the symptom pattern (onset, duration, intensity)? How does event familiarity impact uncertainty? ■ How familiar is the person with the health care environment, rules and routines, and event congruency?
Calls for Nursing ■ What strategies (coping mobilization, affect control, and coping buffering) impact a person's adaptation?
What nursing interventions decrease uncertainty in illness? ■ How can I measure the impact of nursing intervention on the patient's level of uncertainty? ■ What scales developed to measure uncertainty have supported multiple nursing intervention studies and enhanced our understanding of patient behaviors and the impact of clinical nursing practice? ■ How does research related to uncertainty in illness inform my nursing interventions?

(continued)

TABLE 4.9   Guiding Questions: Theory of Uncertainty in Illness (*continued*)

Nursing Outcome To what extent has the person grown to a new value system? ■ What modifications in coping mobilization and affect–control strategies were needed to decrease uncertainty and support growth?

Source: Mishel (1988).

REFERENCES

Boykin, A., & Schoenhofer, S. (1993). *Nursing as caring: A model for transforming practice*. New York, NY: National League for Nursing Press.

Boykin, A., & Schoenhofer, S. (2001). *Nursing as caring: A model for transforming practice*. Boston, MA: Jones & Bartlett Publishers.

Boykin, A., Schoenhofer, S., & Linden, D. (2010). Anne Boykin and Savina Schoenhofer's nursing as caring theory. In M. E. Parker & M. C. Smith (Eds.), *Nursing theories & nursing practice* (3rd ed., pp. 370–386). Philadelphia, PA: F.A. Davis.

Diekelmann, N. (1990). Nursing education: Caring, dialogue, and practice. *Journal of Nursing Education, 29*(7), 300–305.

Florida Atlantic University, Christine E. Lynn College of Nursing. (2012). *Philosophy*. Retrieved from http://nursing.fau.edu/index.php?main=1&nav=635

Hartweg, D., & Fleck, L. (2010). Dorthea Orem's self-care deficit theory. In M. E. Parker & M. C. Smith (Eds.), *Nursing theories & nursing practice* (3rd ed., pp. 121–145). Philadelphia, PA: F.A. Davis.

Helson, H. (1964). *Adaption-level theory*. New York, NY: Harper & Row.

King, B., Barry, C., & Gordon, S. (2014). Lived experience of teaching/learning from nursing situations: A phenomenological study [Abstract]. *International Journal for Human Caring, 18*(3), 88.

Kolcaba, K. (2010). Katherine Kolcaba's comfort theory. In M. E. Parker & M. C. Smith (Eds.), *Nursing theories & nursing practice* (3rd ed., pp. 389–401). Philadelphia, PA: F.A. Davis.

Leininger, M. (1991). *Culture care diversity and universality: A theory of nursing*. New York, NY: National League for Nursing Press.

Leininger, M. M. (2002). Part I: Selected research findings from the culture care theory. In M. M. Leininger & M. R. McFarland (Eds.), *Transcultural nursing: Concepts, theories, and practice* (3rd ed., pp. 99–116). New York, NY: McGraw-Hill.

Leininger, M., & McFarland, M. R. (2010). Madeline Leininger's theory of culture care diversity and universality. In M. Parker & M. Smith (Eds.), *Nursing theory and nursing practice* (3rd ed., pp. 317–336). Philadelphia, PA: F.A. Davis.

Mayeroff, M. (1971). *On caring*. New York, NY: Harper & Row.

Mishel, M. H. (1988). Uncertainty in illness. *Image: Journal of Nursing Scholarship, 20*(4), 225–231.

Mishel, M. H., & Clayton, M. F. (2008). Theories of uncertainty in illness. In M. J. Smith & P. R. Leihr (Eds.), *Middle range theory for nursing* (2nd ed., pp. 55–84). New York, NY: Springer.

Orem, D. (1991). *Nursing: Concepts of practice* (4th ed.). St. Louis, MO: Mosby-Year Book.

Orem, D. (2001). *Nursing: Concept of practice* (6th ed.). St. Louis, MO: Mosby.

Parker, M. E., & Smith, M. C. (2010). A guide for the study of theories for practice. In M. E. Parker & M. C. Smith (Eds.), *Nursing theories & nursing practice* (3rd ed., pp. 16–19). Philadelphia, PA: F.A. Davis.

Roach, M. S. (1987/2002). *Caring, the human mode of being: A blueprint for the health professions (2nd rev. ed)*. Ottawa, Canada: The Canadian Hospital Association Press.

Roach, M. S. (2002). *The human act of caring: A blueprint for the health professions*. Ottawa, Canada: The Canadian Hospital Association Press.

Roy, C. (2009). *The Roy adaptation model* (3rd ed.). Upper Saddle River, NJ: Prentice-Hall Health.

Roy, C., & Zhan, L. (2010). Sister Callista Roy's adaptation model. In M. E. Parker & M. C. Smith (Eds.), *Nursing theories & nursing practice* (3rd ed., pp. 167–181). Philadelphia, PA: F.A. Davis.

Smith, M. C. (2008). Evaluation of middle range theories for the discipline of nursing. In M. J. Smith & P. R. Leihr (Eds.), *Middle range theory for nursing* (2nd ed., pp. 293–314). New York, NY: Springer Publishing.

Smith, M. J., & Liehr, P. R. (2008). *Middle range theory for nursing* (2nd ed.). New York, NY: Springer Publishing.

Touhy, T., & Boykin, A. (2008). Caring as the central domain in nursing. *International Journal for Human Caring, 12*(2), 9–15.

von Bertalanffy, L. (1968). *General systems theory. Foundations, development, applications*. New York, NY: George Braziller.

Watson, J. (2008). *Nursing: The philosophy and science of caring* (2nd rev ed. with Caritas Meditation CD). Boulder, CO: University of Colorado Press.

Watson, J., & Woodward, T. K. (2010). Jean Watson's theory of human caring. In M. E. Parker & M. C. Smith (Eds.), *Nursing theories & nursing practice* (3rd ed., pp. 351–369). Philadelphia, PA: F.A. Davis.

Young, L. B. (1986). *The unfinished universe*. New York, NY: Simon & Schuster.

CHAPTER 5

Exemplar Using a Nursing Situation to Facilitate Teaching/Learning in a Graduate Course on the Discipline of Nursing

Savina O. Schoenhofer

This chapter presents an exemplar of the usefulness of a nursing situation as the focus point to teach the discipline of nursing in a graduate course. One particular nursing situation, titled, "The 4th of July Picnic," is studied as the student responds to assignments throughout the course. Included in this chapter are descriptions of the faculty and student interactions, communications between faculty and student, and development of synthesis of meaning for each. This same nursing situation appears in Chapter 14 for use with undergraduate and graduate students.

COURSE: THE PHILOSOPHICAL AND THEORETICAL DIMENSION OF NURSING AS A PRACTICE DISCIPLINE

COURSE OVERVIEW

Written by Savina O. Schoenhofer, PhD, RN

Michael Shaw told in written form the awe-inspiring story of his nursing a group of men hospitalized with chronic mental illness. He wrote the story in response to an assignment in a beginning graduate course in nursing.

The focus of the course was the philosophical and theoretical dimensions of nursing as a practice discipline. Three learning activities (brief application papers) provided opportunity to examine broad themes in the context of a meaningful personal experience of nursing practice: characteristics of disciplines, philosophy of nursing practice, and a selected extant grand nursing theoretical perspective. The content from Michael's three papers provides the basis for the following analysis.

Directions: Reflect on a nursing situation from practice in which the caring between the nurse and the one nursed enhanced the personhood of the nurse and one nursed.

4TH OF JULY PICNIC

Written by Michael Shaw, BSN, RN

Around the 4th of July, our large hospital provides a dazzling fireworks display for the local community. Everyone is invited and it is a fun-filled event geared toward employees, their families, and our patients. I wanted to do something special for the remaining eight patients that made up the psychiatric ward where I worked. This particular ward was being phased out and these eight men were considered "placement issues" because of the severity of their mental illness. The problem was, I work the A shift and the fireworks show was obviously scheduled in the evening. I began planning a party for the aforementioned men but, because of prior holiday commitments by the staff, found little support for my "party." Undaunted, I proceeded with my plans, eventually soliciting a few dollars.

At 7:00 p.m. the night of the celebration, I showed up with 10 large pizzas, five ice-cold watermelons, a cooler filled with soft drinks, lawn chairs, eight of the coolest-looking straw hats purchased at the local dollar store, and a boom-box with a Michael Jackson CD. We promptly set up folding tables in an open space outside the porch area of our ward that afforded an unobstructed view of the upcoming fireworks.

Let me just say we partied! The eight patients, three staff members, and I had a night to remember! The smiles on everyone's faces as we ate slice after slice of pizza and watermelon and danced to Michael Jackson hits remains a priceless memory. As I surveyed the scene, I was overcome by the feeling that this was more like a family reunion—we weren't just patients and staff members, but friends truly enjoying this special evening together.

Later, as darkness descended upon the grounds, a contented hush fell over our gathering in anticipation of the fireworks slated to begin. The show began, and besides the booming of the fireworks the only sound heard were the *ooohhs* and *aaaahhs* in appreciation of the fireworks that illuminated the evening sky.

Days later our ward would be closed and the patients dispersed, never to be seen or heard from again. As time passed, the glow of that wonderful evening would diminish and I would be transferred to another ward. Then one day as I was searching for an item in a storage closet, I happened across a funky little straw hat and the memories of that dancing while waiting for the fireworks to begin. Nursing is creating positive memories for your patients!

ANALYSIS OF MICHAEL SHAW'S NURSING SITUATION

What Were the Expressions of Caring Between Nurse and the One Being Nursed?

We were present not as just staff members and patients, but as friends gathered for a party; we were there to serve, but not to order or direct our patients as we often do during the course of a normal work day. Also, we were not in uniform, which further broke down the divide between staff and patients. Actually, we were dressed in Hawaiian shirts and straw hats. We laughed and joked with our patients, even dancing with them or for them. The antiseptic atmosphere of their daily routine was replaced with one of relaxation and fun! Even the food we brought added to the festivities. Our patients rarely get to choose what they eat, especially different kinds of real pizza or sodas. "Can I have another one of those real Cokes?" asked one of our contented patients. Little things we take for granted were offered that evening to our party-goers. You should have seen the delight on their faces when we cut open several chilled watermelons. We had a blast with a seed spitting contest! We allowed ourselves to be free with our friends, unencumbered without the responsibility of observing, charting, monitoring, and so on.

What Was the Caring Between the Nurse and the One Nursed?

We focused our efforts to allow these special men a chance to really enjoy themselves just as if they were outside our facility's walls at home. They could be loud, silly, eat as much as they wanted, dance—whatever they wanted to do as long as they didn't harm themselves or others. It was their night!

What Can We Come to Know That Will Help Us Understand the Call for Nursing in This Situation?

Remember why most of us got into nursing? It might sound cliché, but yeah, "I want to make a difference! Help people!" That's what we experienced that wonderful evening! Oh, the drudgery that sometimes make up our days as nurses—the meetings, the audits, in-services—but then, at any patient encounter, one can choose to make a difference! A smile, or kind word, just listening quietly to a concerned patient goes a tremendous way—and it is so simple to do! Never lose sight of what we are called to do! Remember receiving your first nursing degree, how excited we were, you were ready to conquer the world…we acted like new nurses that evening!

Insights

- We were equals that night.
- These lonely men felt like being part of a caring family for the first time in a long time.
- The feelings of being institutionalized evaporated for those few brief hours.
- Someone cared, someone responded to a need.
- The unselfish, kind acts of the staff that showed up that night! I'm still in awe.
- What a tremendous change in attitudes that occurred among the participants that evening.

ASSIGNMENT 1: CHARACTERISTICS OF DISCIPLINES

From King and Brownell's (1976) characteristics of disciplines, Michael selected three that resonated particularly well with his nursing situation: imagination, community, and caring as a valuative and affective stance.

Imagination

Drawing on Le Sorti and colleagues' (1999) call for creative thinking in nursing, Michael wrote that "an after-hours party for a few challenged, sequestered men is practically unheard of, yet falls squarely into that call for creativity." Conceptualizing, planning, and carrying out the 4th of July picnic was recognized in Michael's paper as an expression of "formation and production of a novel and meaningful idea or product" (p. 62) that characterizes imaginative nursing practice.

Community

Michael quoted a classic work on the power of friendship in long-term care institutions, asserting that they should be encouraged to "compensate for the loss of virtually all pre-existing relationships" (Miller & Beer, 1977), and added, "This profoundly describes the patients for whom our party was given…we were their only community…the only family they could count on. We became their friends." Here, Michael drew on Geanellos (2002), who explained that when nurses are friendly, patients' feelings of comfort, belonging, and involvement increase. In a later conversation Michael told me, "We were just friends having a party; it was like a neighborhood block party!"

Caring

Michael asked the question, "Who cared if these men missed another party? They were never invited before and probably would not even be aware of the ongoing festivities." Finfgeld-Connett's (2008) concept of caring as a component of nursing-guiding paradigm was recognized in relation to caring as a valuative and affective stance in nursing. Further, Michael confirmed Finfgeld-Connett's view that caring has the potential to improve the well-being of patients and nurses when he said, "It certainly did on that one summer evening for the patients and staff assembled there; as it turned out, both the patients and this nurse were beneficiaries of this event."

ASSIGNMENT 2: PHILOSOPHY AND NURSING PRACTICE

The second application paper was built on the study of the concept of paradigm, from the perspective of Guba's (1990) four paradigms. Michael decided that the paradigm most closely reflecting his worldview was constructivism. Constructivism was selected through a process of elimination, based largely on his preference for freedom and creativity. He recognized that it was his intention to provide an opportunity for the hospitalized men in his group, each of whom had a unique reality, to participate and enjoy themselves freely. Michael concluded his brief paper by noting, "Nursing requires open-mindedness"—where creativity can be embraced and each is permitted his own subjectivity.

ASSIGNMENT 3: SELECTED EXTANT NURSING THEORETICAL PERSPECTIVE

Michael selected Jean Watson's Theory of Human Caring as the broad theoretical lens that gives shape to his approach to nursing practice. In particular, he selected two concepts—Fox's *via* and Watson's *caritas* processes—as focal lenses for his broad theoretical understanding of the nursing situation.

The *Via*

The *via negativa* requires one to "show up and choose to be present" (Watson, 2000), acknowledging the dark and the light. A party like Michael planned had not been done before in that place and held potential risks; nonetheless, upset that this group of men weren't invited to join in the celebration, he determined that something had to be done. So he planned a real party, with straw hats for all; pizzas, Cokes, and watermelon; a boom box and dancing; staff members in Hawaiian shirts—in other words, he and his staff colleagues showed up and chose to be present to their intentions. Michael reported that as the evening progressed, "we transitioned onto the next path, the *via positiva*," the path that brings forth light and a positive loving caring energy. In Michael's words, "Surveying this splendid scene, all one could see and hear were the smiles and laughter as men danced, ate and morphed into a family unit enjoying a reunion-like atmosphere." He told me in a later conversation, "We were all brothers."

Caritas Processes

Applying the lens of Watson's caritas processes to the study of this nursing situation, Michael chose "the practice of loving kindness and equanimity" (Watson & Woodward, 2010) to illustrate that the barriers between staff and patients were dismantled. He explained, "The fellowship we shared characterized yet another caritas process, that of developing and sustaining a helping–trusting caring relationship" (2010). A third caritas process "brought to life that evening involved the creative use of self as part of the caring process...a transpersonal moment in which staff and patients sparked a connection with each other." Michael continued, "There under the stars and between brilliant flashes of fireworks booming overhead, a caring–healing–loving consciousness was formed." When the fireworks and party were over, Michael reports that he "witnessed something very special, a column of men with arms around shoulders, giggling, laughing, and, yes, even belching as they brought this magical evening to a close." Michael concluded, "We freed ourselves to allow love and caring to come together (Watson, 1998), we were not machines but spirit made whole" (Watson, 2003).

APPLICATION OF THE BARRY, GORDON & KING TEACHING/LEARNING NURSING FRAMEWORK BY DR. SAVINA SCHOENHOFER

What Were the Expressions of Caring Between Nurse and the One Nursed?

Michael has shared his understanding of the expressions of caring in his nursing situation. The nurse directly participating in the *caring between* in real time has special knowledge of the caring that was lived between nurse and one nursed. However, as the nursing situation is being engaged as an open text, others can participate and contribute to the growing shared understanding of expressions of caring in this situation. This leads to an enriched appreciation of the nursing situation at hand and of other situations that share characteristics, and even possibly touching on the very heart of all nursing situations in a meaningful way. This discussion illustrates some of how I participated with Michael in the study and appreciation of nursing, through the medium of his nursing situation. My role as course facilitator was to provide content for some of the key ideas in the course, to create learning activities intended to promote deep learning at personal and theoretical levels, and to participate in the online dialogue with Michael and other students. In addition, after the conclusion of the course, I invited Michael to dialogue with me to help me more fully picture the nursing situation and its meaning to him and the other direct participants. In my analysis, I will offer my own insight into aspects of the situation, recognizing that it may coincide or offer an alternative view with the insight gained by Michael and with anyone else sharing in the study of this nursing situation at any past or future time. My purpose here is to explore the meaning of the nursing situation from my own experience, with part of that experience being my access to and participation in Michael's written and verbal sharing of the situation. It is not intended that any suggested meanings are the "best" or "final" meaning. That is part of the value of studying nursing situations in this way—it is always possible, and likely, for new meaning to emerge, suggesting new ways of practice.

Roach's Caring Entailments

- *Compassion*: Michael and his staff colleagues felt compassion for the men entrusted in their care, recognizing that these men were part of the community and deserved to be included in the community celebration. Michael also felt compassion for his staff colleagues, saying "it warmed my heart that four members of the staff showed up after hours" to participate in the party.
- *Conscience*: Michael said, on learning that the men in his group were being excluded from the 4th of July celebration shared by the hospital and surrounding community, "something had to be done."
- *Competence*: Michael used his knowledge of the hospital system and his social skills to secure permission for the unprecedented special party, and then organized all the components of a real July 4th celebration.
- *Confidence*: Michael proceeded with plans, trusting that he could make it work and that the party would be a worthwhile experience for all.
- *Commitment*: Michael "sent forth" his conscientious compassionate intention, seeing it through, not being deterred by the dark side of the *via negative*, but choosing to enact his way of caring for the men in his group, thus "comporting" himself in a way that was beautifully congruent with his values, intentions, knowledge, and skill.

Mayeroff's Caring Ingredients

- *Knowing*: As an ingredient of caring in this nursing situation, knowing self and knowing and recognizing other as one with self, a shared humanity, played a key role.
- *Patience*: Michael, other staff colleagues, and patients all demonstrated patience with the idea of making a party. A sense of active patience seemed to be reflected by Michael as he planned and organized. All participants seem to reflect Mayeroff's allusion to patience as tolerance of a certain amount of confusion and floundering as they undertook an activity unique to their experience.
- *Alternating rhythm*: Michael's use of the *via negativa* and *via positiva* in understanding the situation is an example of this caring ingredient. In addition, as the planner/coordinator of the event and simultaneously an active party-goer, Michael expressed alternating rhythm in overseeing the details while sharing in the joy of the moment.
- *Humility*: All party-goers expressed caring for self and other by participation in the event, demonstrating acceptance that there is always more to learn about self and others and caring. It involved an acceptance of both limitations and powers. An important aspect of caring that Mayeroff (1971) discusses under the ingredient of humility is the realization that one's particular way of caring is not in any way privileged; Michael openly expressed the willingness to appreciate each party-goer's way of participating in the festivities.
- *Hope*: An appreciation of the "plentitude of the present, a present alive with the sense of the possible" (Mayeroff, 1971, p. 32)—Michael's description of the shared joy of participation lets us know that hope was very much alive in the hearts of all the participants.
- *Trust*: Mayeroff describes trust as "appreciating the independent existence of the other" (p. 29), and other *as* other, allowing opportunities for growth. In Michael's paper on philosophy and nursing practice, he addressed open-mindedness and respect for subjectivity, elements that reflect the caring ingredient of trust.
- *Honesty*: Mayeroff says that honesty as caring involves seeing truly. Although we can only hypothesize about other participants' readiness to "see truly," it is clear that Michael has that willingness when he says that his duty that summer day was to see that the men in his group realized their own subjective reality by "allowing them to participate and express their own enjoyment as they perceived fit."
- *Courage*: "Taking heart," risking, and courage clearly were ways of caring that were actively lived by all participants, simply in their being there and being themselves, in authentic presence.

The Caring Between

From the perspective of the theory of nursing as caring, the *caring between* is the space within which nursing is created. After studying Michael's written story and analysis, I invited him to have a conversation with me about the caring between in the situation. For him, the caring between was experienced as letting barriers down and having fun together, like brothers, like a family reunion, like a neighborhood block party. His emphasis on the barrier-free relating, the elimination of barriers presented by role, and by expectations based on previous behavior led me to a sense of the essence of the caring between all participants as "sharing normalcy."

Using the Ways of Knowing, How Can We Come to Understand the Call(s) for Nursing?

Personal knowing: Has Michael experienced feeling left out, being not wanted, or has he witnessed the experience of another being left out that has attuned him to this situation? Perhaps. I have personally experienced and witnessed being left out and can easily relate to Michael's awareness that the men in his group were left out of the 4th of July festivities. From early childhood playground days, there are opportunities to at least sense the pain and sadness of those "picked last" for teams and of the sense of inequity often felt by all involved.

Empirical knowing: Social psychological theories of the human experience of inclusion and exclusion, social stigma, and therapeutic community contribute to empirical knowing for this situation. In Michael's paper on community as a characteristic of nursing as a discipline, he addressed the empirical benefits of inclusion and belongingness, citing three sources from gerontology and nursing. A broad range of research and theory could contribute to empirical knowing in studying this story.

Ethical knowing: Michael demonstrated the impact of ethical knowing in his statement, related to the failure of the men in his group to be invited to the 4th of July festivities, that "something had to be done." Awareness of the need for action, and specifically for *right action*, is central to ethical knowing.

Aesthetic knowing: Michael's vision of a genuine 4th of July picnic as an expression of family and community was the early spark for the nursing situation. In communicating with Michael over the course of the semester and beyond, I am aware of a marvelous evolution of understanding of nursing as a creative art and of himself as nurse artist, through the pathway of aesthetic knowing. As I look back to the summary statement of the essence of caring in his nursing situation, expressed in the beginning of the semester as, "Nursing is creating positive memories for your patients!" and recollect one of his last statements to me ("all barriers were down"; "the smiles and joy of a reunion"), aesthetic knowing has continued to bear fruit.

Sociopolitical knowing, unknowing, and emancipatory knowing: These pathways of knowing converged in Michael's observation that "Nursing requires the open mindedness of constructivism, where individuals can construct their own reality, and subjectivity is embraced." A great deal more could be said here, but the quote from Michael's paper can provide the stimulus for future reflection on the role of these ways of knowing in his situation.

What Are the Calls for Nursing?

How can we express the central call for nursing in this situation? The Theory of Nursing as Caring proposes that a call for caring in nursing is an explicit situated form of the universal call to "know me now as caring person and affirm me…a call for acknowledgement and affirmation of living caring in specific ways in this situation" (Boykin & Schoenhofer, 2001, p. 13).

What Were the Responses to the Calls for Nursing in the Situation?

To clearly identify responses to calls for nursing—calls for caring in nursing—a clear notion of the unifying call needs to be made explicit. As I mentioned earlier, there is no one way to answer the question, "What is the call for nursing?" in any given situation. The coming together of the nurse, one nursed, and circumstances always presents a unique nursing situation and, at the same time, the unique nursing situation presented is a reflection of any and all nursing situations. It is the universality dimension of the nursing situation that renders it an exquisite open text for the study of nursing. In conversation with Michael, I expressed my grasp of the call for caring in his nursing situation as a call for celebrating shared normalcy. Michael readily agreed that celebrating shared normalcy was a useful representation of the call for nursing in his nursing situation. This understanding of the call is the basis for identifying responses to that call.

In Paterson and Zderad's (2007) *Humanistic Nursing*, it is made clear that both nurse and patient are calling and responding simultaneously as well as in alternating rhythm. *Calling* and *responding* are terms that celebrate openness and viability, mutuality and creativity. *Call* and *response* are terms that seem more static, more fixed, though suitable for use in identifying *outcomes* of nurse caring as *products* of nursing. Both sets of terms can be useful in *thinking nursing* in situations. The gerund form (calling and responding) respects the dynamic nature of nursing as a shared human relationship, whereas the noun form (call and response) permits the generation of reasonable and necessary accountability standards. I will attempt to address both forms in discussing responses to the call for caring in this nursing situation and, subsequently, in the discussion of outcomes.

Drawing on all patterns of knowing, Michael empathized with the men in his care group being excluded from the community celebration, and he responded to the call for celebrating shared normalcy initially by deciding to facilitate a party. Michael also called out to his staff colleagues to join in this caring call for sharing normalcy, and to Michael's delight three of the staff showed up, off the clock, to take part. Other responses described in the story came from the surrounding community: permission to hold the party and funds made available.

As with many stories of nursing situations, there are missing details that require the student of the story to generalize and to reach out through multiple ways of knowing and hypothesize. In Michael's story, the details we do have suggest that the men of the care unit did not explicitly call for celebrating shared normalcy, such that Michael's response in creating the party was an obvious answer to the call. So the question arises—What *was* the source of the call? The noted nursing theorist Dorothea Orem (1985) answered this question in relation to her own theoretical concept, self-care deficit. Her answer was that the self-care deficit (or, in our case, the call) was formed in the mind of the nurse (Orem, 1985). Ideally, a call for nursing is understood by the nurse as an integration of all that is known of the situation, expressed in a language that provides a justifiable central focus for accountable nursing action. Sometimes stories of nursing situations contain direct evidence of calls for caring, but often there is no direct confirmation from the patient that the nurse's formulation of the call for caring was on target. In practice guided by the nursing as caring theory, nurses extend a direct invitation for those nursed to express and clarify their call for caring. An example of this direct invitation is: How may I care for you today in ways that matter to you?

However, in studying nursing by using stories of nursing situations as text, the "one right understanding" is not only unnecessary, it constitutes a barrier to the learner's creativity and expanded understanding. In Michael's story, we lack detailed evidence that would lend confirmation of the call from patients. However, based on my experience of working with nurses, helping them to make the tacit explicit, I am confident that Michael could provide details that would provide support for the call for caring formulated as "celebrating shared normalcy." With that confidence comes permission to associate patient response with nurse caring. The active, ebullient participation of the patients—getting into the party mode, dancing, enjoying the food and drink, smiling and talking freely and naturally, the arms around shoulders as they left the party to return to the hospital building—demonstrates the responses of the nursed to nurse caring in this situation.

What Was the Outcome of the Response?

There are several questions that could be asked to clarify and direct this discussion of outcomes of nurse caring. One question that is important in relation to supportability of outcome determinations is: What was the response to the response? Another is: What is the further call for caring implied in the response, and in the response to the response? Yet another question is: What value was experienced in a nursing situation (Schoenhofer & Boykin, 1998)? These questions relate to my earlier discussion of call–response and calling–responding. One dimension of the concept of nursing situation is accountability. A statement of outcome refers to a somewhat arbitrary and preferably agreed-upon stopping point in determining what counts as nursing, and the value of that which counts as nursing. In other words, outcome statements are cause-and-effect representations of what came about in and through the nursing situation. This kind of point-in-time assessment is one legitimate aspect of nursing practice. In addition, there is another dimension of the nursing situation that calls, not for accounting, but for creating and appreciating the open dynamic nature of the practice and discipline of nursing. Realizing these two distinct dimensions is a way of speaking to caring for the discipline and practice itself through the dynamic of alternating rhythm.

Although it is important to establish the value of nurse caring in situations, it is also worthwhile to extend that assessment beyond the nurse–nursed, reaching out into the larger space of the nursing situation. An example of this kind of accounting for the value of nurse caring is described in Schoenhofer and Boykin's (1998) study of a nursing situation that occurred in a rural community. Not only were assessments of value experienced through the nursing situation offered by the nurse practitioner and the one nursed, but also by the nursing director and by the CEO of the home health agency involved. In addition, monetary values were calculated where feasible.

As a foundation for assessing outcomes of nurse caring in Michael's nursing situation or any other, it is necessary to be clear about the theoretical perspective that frames the concepts of nursing, nurse caring, and outcomes of nurse caring. An economic model as the foundation for outcomes assessment will produce insight about the economics relevant to the nursing situation. A medical model framework will address only those aspects of nurse caring and outcomes of nurse caring that relate to the medically directed aspects of the situation. For congruence and coherence, the nursing model that frames an assessment of the value of nursing in a situation should be explicit and the design and implementation of care should have been framed on that same nursing model. My discussion of outcomes of nurse caring in Michael's nursing situation is framed from the theoretical perspective of nursing as caring (Boykin & Schoenhofer, 2001). That theoretical perspective calls for descriptions of the value experienced within the nursing situation.

For the ones nursed: The value experienced through the nursing situation by the men in the care unit has to be projected based on data provided by Michael and assumptions gained through the various patterns of knowing. Michael's description of the scene lets us be reasonably confident in saying that those men valued the experience of celebrating shared normalcy. Their enthusiastic participation in the partying and the image of them joining a column of men with walking back to the unit with arms around each other's shoulders add to our confidence in drawing the conclusion that Michael's expressions of caring in response to the intuited call for celebrating shared normalcy were effective in contributing to enhanced personhood. Another possible bit of evidence that the call was effectively answered is that Michael has not reported any problem behavior. In fact, he expressed astonishment to me that these men—who routinely yell, curse, and spit at staff and each other—are, in his words, "just wonderful people who wanted to have a good time."

For the nurse: Michael's statements, on paper and in conversation, give clear evidence upon which to assess the value of the nursing situation to him. His sense of nurse as creative artist, his realization of nursing as artistry and a forum for creativity, were awakened and confirmed through the experience of the nursing situation. His willingness to care, to hear an unusual call for caring, and to take novel steps to respond to that call have strengthened his confidence in nursing and himself. He was moved that staff members came through despite early disinterest; based on what Michael has written, his sense of the care team as family, as persons he can count on, has been strengthened. Michael has grown in personhood through the value experienced in the nursing situation. Personhood, that is, living grounded in caring, was reconfirmed and enhanced through the experience of caring between him, the staff members, and the patients. He has continued to grow in personhood, as nurse, through sharing his story and reflecting on it through new lenses.

For the staff: Members of the staff who came to the party off the clock no doubt found value in the experience of the nursing situation as they responded to Michael's call for support; through their presence, they responded as well to the call for celebrating shared normalcy. It is possible that they have gained an increased sense of the value of authentic presence—with colleagues and with patients. It is reasonable to assume that they value the example provided by Michael's courageous, loving initiative to take action that is needed even though unconventional.

For the health care system: To extend consideration of outcomes to the health care setting is important, even though in this situation we will be projecting possible values to be experienced in the health care system itself. One value is the enhancement of staff vision and capacities. The strength and maturity gained by Michael and the other participating staff is a valuable asset to the institution. Another potential outcome of this nursing situation could be a realization by the leaders of the health care system that ways could and should be found to include all members of the community in future important events.

For others: We could extend the circle of the nursing situation to include the surrounding community, the state mental health department, and the larger society. Where large complex systems are a key feature of the study of nursing situations, this can and should be done. Part of the larger social matrix that has gained value from participating in the study of Michael's nursing situation includes the graduate class in which he shared his story. In the online dialogue for the class, classmates and teacher shared appreciation for Michael's nursing and were inspired by his creativity and initiative, as well as by his commitment to living the meaning of caring in his everyday life.

OTHER LEADINGS

The discussion and analysis of the story of Michael's nursing situation are only beginning illustrations of the way this story could be used to enrich the study of nearly any nursing topic. Both Michael and I have worked within the structure of the story, with its details, in our discussion. However, the story could and should be the basis for a more extensive study of nursing, employing a wide range of variations of detail and theory.

REFERENCES

Boykin, A., & Schoenhofer, S. O. (2001). *Nursing as caring: A model for transforming practice.* Sudbury, MA: Jones & Bartlett. Retrieved from http://www.gutenberg.org/ebooks/42988

Finfgeld-Connett, D. (2008). Meta-synthesis of caring in nursing. *Journal of Clinical Nursing, 17*(2), 196–204. doi:10.1111/j.1365-270.2006.0184.x

Geanellos, R. (2002). Exploring the therapeutic potential of friendliness and friendship in nursing-client relationships. *Contemporary Nurse, 12*(3), 235–245. doi:10.5172/conu.12.3.235

Guba, E. C. (1990). *The alternative paradigm dialog.* In E. C. Guba (Ed.), *The paradigm dialog* (pp. 17–27). Newbury Park, CA: Sage Publications.

King, A., & Brownell, J. (1976). *The curriculum and the disciplines of knowledge.* Huntington, NY: Robert E. Krieger Publishing Company.

Le Sorti, A. J., Cullen, P. A., Hanzlik, E. M., Michiels, J. M., Piano, L. A., Ryan, P. L., & Johnson, W. (1999). Creative thinking in nursing education preparing for tomorrow's challenges. *Nursing Outlook, 47*(2), 62–66.

Mayeroff, M. (1971). *On caring.* New York, NY: Harper & Row.

Miller, D. B., & Beer, S. (1977). Patterns of friendship among patients in a nursing home setting. *The Gerontologist, 17*(3), 269–275.

Orem, D. E. (1985). *Nursing: Concepts of practice* (3rd ed.). New York, NY: McGraw-Hill.

Paterson, J., & Zderad, L. (2007). *Humanistic nursing.* Retrieved from http://www.gutenberg.org/files/25020/25020-8.txt

Schoenhofer, S., & Boykin, A. (1998). The value of caring experienced in nursing. *International Journal for Human Caring, 2*(4), 9–15.

Watson, J. (1998). *Theories of human caring.* Retrieved from http://watsoncaringscience.org/about-us/caring-science-definitions-processes-theory/

Watson, J. (2000). Leading via caring-healing: The four-fold way toward transformative leadership. *Nursing Administration Quarterly, 25*(1), 1–6.

Watson, J. (2003). Love and caring: Ethics of face and hand—an invitation to return to the heart and soul of nursing and our deep humanity. *Nursing Administration Quarterly, 27*(3), 197–202.

Watson, J., & Woodward, T. K. (2010). Jean Watson's theory of human caring. In M. E. Parker & M. C. Smith (Eds.), *Nursing theories and nursing practice* (3rd ed., pp. 351–369). Philadelphia, PA: F. A. Davis Company.

PART II

Nursing Situation Exemplars

CHAPTER 6

Caring Between the Nurse and an Older Adult in an ER

This chapter presents a nursing situation focused on caring for an older man presenting in the emergency room for evaluation of a possible cerebral vascular accident (stroke). Using the philosophical perspective of caring (FAU, CON, 2012), which focuses on nurturing the wholeness and well-being of persons in caring relationships, the nursing situation highlights the aesthetic response to a call for nursing to provide hopeful, authentic presence as the patient and wife await test results in an intense emergency room.

Directions: As you prepare to intentionally enter the world of the other, reflect on the following question: What are the expressions of caring between nurse and the one nursed?

NURSING SITUATION

Written by Alana Andrews, BSN, RN

REALISTIC HOPEFULNESS

"This patient to room one!" I hear my charge nurse yell out. In our emergency department, room one is our most high acuity room, which we reserve for cardiac arrests and high acuity patients. The patient is an older man, maybe in his mid-60s. He has gray, short hair and fair skin. His eyes are closed and he looks calm, almost as though sleeping. I hear "Code Sert" announced over the intercom and realize the patient in front of me is possibly having a stroke.

Emergency rooms are always a flurry of activity and commotion but even more so during a "Code" of any sort. I immediately begin assessing, taking vital signs, and drawing blood from Mr. Edwards, my patient in room one. He opens his eyes minimally for me, answers some of my questions, and tries to follow the numerous commands I give him. His entire left side is flaccid, including a left side facial droop. His speech is slurred and somewhat delayed. An ED technician and I rush Mr. Edwards out of the department to CT scan. We place him on the table for his brain scan and, for the first time, I see he is staring at me, wide-eyed and anxious. I explain what the test is and why we need to do it immediately. Mr. Edwards nods ever so slightly and I squeeze his shoulder. I look straight into his eyes and whisper, "It's going to be okay."

As we walk back into room one with Mr. Edwards on our stretcher, I see a tiny older woman standing against the wall. Her eyes are glistened over with tears. In her hands she holds a handkerchief and a rosary wrapped around her fingers. Without a word, she walks to his side and takes his limp hand in hers and they both look toward me. I wanted to look away or leave the room but I knew in this moment these two people needed me. I walked over to him and took his other hand. I slowly and clearly explained that the doctors believed Mr. Edwards was having a stroke. I described what the CT scan would show and how we may treat him depending on the results. "What do we do until the results come back?" Mrs. Edwards asked me. "We just wait," I answered. Mr. Edwards looked up at his wife's face and one small tear ran down his cheek. I felt so lost. I didn't know how to comfort them and I couldn't leave them. Mrs. Edwards suddenly stood up straight, took my hand in hers, and said, "We will wait and we will hope. We will hope for everything to be alright. We will hope for answers. In this time when we have no cards to play, we will just hope."

Mrs. Edwards taught me a lesson that night. She taught me something no professor, textbook, or course ever could. She taught me the lesson of hope and the true power of hope in times of need. In those minutes of waiting, our emotional bond grew as did Mr. Edwards's resolve to live. Mr. Edwards ended up receiving a tissue plasminogen activator (tPA) that night to dissolve the clot in his brain. His symptoms were mostly resolved by the next morning. I will never forget Mr. and Mrs. Edwards and the idea they have inspired. The essence of caring in this nursing situation is *hope*.

STUDY PROCESS

The Barry, Gordon & King Teaching/Learning Nursing Framework process is a broad guide to study and analyze nursing situations, focusing on the caring between the nurse and one nursed. The following analysis guides and inspires understanding of nursing from the *philosophical perspective of caring* (FAU, CON, 2012), focusing on nurturing the wholeness and well-being of persons in caring relationships.

What Was the Caring Between the Nurse and the One Nursed?

The nurse asserts the essence of caring in this nursing situation is hope. What expressions of caring are present in this nursing situation? How did the nurse facilitate hope? What was the value of the nurse staying with Mr. and Mrs. Edwards while waiting for test results?

Using the Ways of Knowing, How Can We Come to Understand the Call(s) for Nursing?

How does each of the ways of knowing—personal, empirical, ethical, sociopolitical, spiritual, emancipatory, unknowing, and aesthetic—inform understanding of caring in this nursing situation (Carper, 1978; Kagen, Smith, Cowling, & Chinn, 2009; Munhall, 1993; White, 1995)?

Personal knowing: What do I know about cerebral vascular accidents? What can I learn from Mr. and Mrs. Edwards about hope while waiting for CT scan results? What have I conveyed as a caring person? How can I be helpful to them? What do I know about supporting Mrs. Edwards?

Empirical knowing: What knowledge is needed to provide nursing care for a person undergoing a series of tests for stroke? What are the standard protocols for care of persons experiencing a stroke? What ongoing nursing assessments are needed? What changes are important to document and convey to all members of the emergency room team? What patient teaching will be needed for a person who experiences a stroke? What medications, dietary restrictions, and need for exercise may be needed to limit neurologic deficits and/or prevent future events? How does hope sustain persons during difficult situations?

Ethical knowing: What ethical issues are present in this nursing situation? How do codes of ethics guide practice?

Sociopolitical knowing: What is the sociological impact of cerebral vascular accidents? How can the nurse support Mr. and Mrs. Edwards as they navigate the health insurance coverage for his hospital stay and tests? How does culture impact Mr. Edwards's understanding of health? How does geographic location influence access to care for persons experiencing a stroke?

Spiritual knowing: What knowledge is needed for the nurse to understand the spiritual impact of experiencing an acute, and possibly devastating, health concern? How can the nurse support Mr. and Mrs. Edwards in their spiritual needs?

Emancipatory knowing: What will it be like for Mr. Edwards to live with neurologic deficits? What bureaucratic barriers may influence Mr. Edwards's recovery and rehabilitation?

Unknowing: What matters most to Mr. Edwards at this moment in time? How was the nurse open to understanding the nursing situation from the perspective of Mr. and Mrs. Edwards? What did the nurse communicate through her actions and communication?

Aesthetic knowing: How did the nurse support this couple's hopes and dreams? How does aesthetic re-presentation of the nursing situation inform nursing?

What Are the Calls for Nursing?

The nurse identified hope, comfort, authentic presence, and alternating rhythms as the calls she heard from Mr. and Mrs. Edwards. What other calls are present in this nursing situation?

What Are the Responses to the Calls for Nursing Present in the Situation?

How did the nurse respond with authentic presence? What expressions of caring are evident as responses to the call for comfort and alternating rhythms?

What Was the Outcome of the Response(s) in Relation to the Call(s)?

The nurse used the philosophical perspective of caring (FAU, CON, 2012), which focuses on nurturing the wholeness and well-being of persons in caring relationships.

In what ways did the outcomes reflect this theoretical lens?

For the person nursed, Mr. Edwards: What mattered most to Mr. Edwards was to stay hopeful while awaiting test results.

For the nurse: The nurse learned the lesson of hope and the true power of hope in times of need.

For the nursing profession: This nursing situation offers an opportunity for nurses to remember the nursing response of hoping for something better in the moment for all persons.

For others: What is the value of being cared for? What is the meaning of hope for a person's well-being? What is the impact of evidence-based interventions on health care costs?

How Did the Study of This Nursing Situation Enhance Your Knowledge of Nursing?

What did I learn about myself as I studied this situation? What did I learn about caring science? What new possibilities can I create from this nursing situation?

LEARNING ACTIVITIES

Journal: Reflect on the courage needed by the nurse bearing witness to the pain and suffering of persons.

BOX 6.1   Reflective Journal

What are your thoughts on caring expressed by the nurse in this situation?

Aesthetic project: Re-presentation by the nurse

BOX 6.2   Aesthetic Re-presentation by the Nurse

This is Alana Andrews's aesthetic re-presentation of her nursing situation.

"Today as I sit and think of hope, I think of all the patients I have cared for and I write for them. I wish to write a poem to soothe their concerns and pull them out of despair. Something simple, perhaps, but [something that] discusses hope in a meaningful way. I am working with my piece to make it look like an ancient manuscript. This aged appearance depicts that humans have known of the power of hope for hundreds of years. Hope is a universal phenomenon that I will now always use with my patients to promote recovery and motivate their rehabilitation."

Hope
Like a stream running down a hill
No knowledge of what lies ahead
Full force and vulnerable, you gush
You slip, you slide
Yet unlike that stream, you worry
You fuss and you fret
What lies ahead! I must know
I cannot go on this way!
Calm your thoughts with quiet resolve
The cool reassuring wave pours over
Hope
Sometimes it's all we possess

Aesthetic project: How can this nursing situation be aesthetically re-presented?

BOX 6.3   Aesthetic Re-presentation

How would you aesthetically re-present this nursing situation?

REFERENCES

Carper, B. (1978). Fundamental patterns of knowing. *Advances in Nursing Science*, *1*(1), 13–24.

Florida Atlantic University, Christine E. Lynn College of Nursing. (2012). *Philosophy*. Retrieved from http://nursing.fau.edu/index.php?main=1&nav=635

Kagen, P. N., Smith, M. C., Cowling, R., & Chinn, P. (2009). A nursing manifesto: An emancipatory call for nursing knowledge development, conscience, and practice. *Nursing Philosophy, 11*, 67–84.

Munhall, P. (1993). Unknowing: Toward another pattern of knowing. *Nursing Outlook, 41*, 125–128.

White, J. (1995). Patterns of knowing: Review, critique, and update. *Advances in Nursing Science, 17*(4), 73–86.

LEARNING RESOURCES

Adeoye, O., Albright, K., Carr, B. G., Wolff, C., Mullen, M. T., Abruzzo, T., . . . Kleindorfer, D. (2014). Geographic access to acute stroke care in the United States. *Stroke, 45*, 3019–3024. doi:10.1161/STROKEAHA.114.006293

Duggleby, W., Cooper, D., & Penz, K. (2009). Hope, self-efficacy, spiritual well-being and job satisfaction. *Journal of Advanced Nursing, 65*(11), 2376–2385. doi:10.111/j.1365-2648.2009.05094.x

Mok, E., Lau, K-P., Lam, W-M., Chan, L-N., Ng, J., & Chan, K. (2010). Healthcare professionals' perceptions of existential distress in patients with advanced cancer. *Journal of Advanced Nursing, 66*(7), 1510–1522. doi:10.1111/j.1365-2648.2010.05330.x

Turner, S. (2005). Hope seen through the eyes of 10 Australian young people. *Journal of Advanced Nursing, 52*(5), 508–517.

Tutton, E., Seers, K., Langstaff, D., & Westwood, M. (2012). Staff and patient views of the concept of hope on a stroke unit: A qualitative study. *Journal of Advanced Nursing, 68*(9), 2061–2069. doi:10.1111/j.1365-2648.2011.05899.x

Caring Between a Nurse and a Young Woman Experiencing a Sickle Cell Crisis in an ER

This chapter presents a nursing situation focused on caring for the emergent emotional and physical needs of a woman experiencing severe pain during a sickle cell crisis. Using the philosophical perspective of caring (FAU, CON, 2012), which focuses on nurturing the wholeness and well-being of persons in caring relationships, the nursing situation highlights response to a call for nursing to provide authentic presence and empathy.

Directions: As you prepare to intentionally enter the world of the other, reflect on the following question: What are the expressions of caring between nurse and the one nursed?

NURSING SITUATION

Written by Molly Johnson, EdS, ASN, RN

HAND SQUEEZE

One afternoon, Ms. Sands, a young woman, was wheeled into one of my assigned rooms in the emergency room (ER). She was moaning, crying, and flailing her arms and legs. I asked her what was happening and she just grunted incoherently. I could see that she was very uncomfortable and agitated. With the help of the medic, we transferred her from the wheelchair to the stretcher still flailing and crying. Ms. Sands reached out and grabbed my hand, squeezing tightly. I told her to take a deep breath and asked, "How can I help?" She took a breath and said she was in a lot of pain in a sickle cell crisis. I asked if she was allergic to any medications and what was her height and weight. Ms. Sands just shook her head and squeezed my hand harder. I kept my focus on her and encouraged her to take slow deep breaths while I instructed the medic to insert an IV. Ms. Sands maintained a tight grip on my right hand.

This was one time I appreciated the small size of the ER room. I was able to take her vital signs and placed a cool wet towel on her sweaty forehead with my left hand as she held on to my right hand. I told her to continue breathing while I propped a blue emesis bag under her chin and changed the wet towel on her forehead. I explained in a soft tone that I needed to leave the room to get some pain medication. I took her hand off mine and placed it on the bed railing. As I turned to leave the room, she asked me to call her sister. She pointed to her purse moaning and flailing her legs intermediately and indicated that her cell phone was in there. Initially I thought calling her sister could wait, but then I considered what I would have wanted if our roles were reversed. So I picked up her purse and gave it to her so she could retrieve her phone. As I opened the phone, I asked her if the name on the screen was her sister's. I called her sister and explained who I was, and that I was calling on behalf of Ms. Sands, who wanted her to know that she was in the ER and she needed her. After hanging up the phone, my patient whispered, "Thank you," and reached out for my hand. I grabbed her hand and squeezed it tightly for about 10 seconds while looking into her eyes. Then I released her hand and left the room to get medication and IV fluids.

Although 15 minutes had gone by, I had only gathered a limited amount of information and I had not documented anything. I followed the lead of the patient, understood her perspective, and addressed her immediate physical and emotional needs. This was a genuine nursing interaction with the focus of care delivered from the patient's perception. The essence of caring in this nursing situation is empathy and authentic presence.

STUDY PROCESS

The Barry, Gordon & King Teaching/Learning Nursing Framework process is a broad guide to study and analyze nursing situations focusing on the caring between the nurse and one nursed. The following analysis guides and inspires understanding of nursing from the philosophical perspective of caring (FAU, CON, 2012), focusing on nurturing the wholeness and well-being of persons in caring relationships.

What Was the Caring Between the Nurse and the One Nursed?

The nurse identified empathy and authentic presence as the essence of caring in this nursing situation. What other expressions of caring are present in this nursing situation?

Using the Ways of Knowing, How Can We Come to Understand the Call(s) for Nursing?

How does each of the ways of knowing—personal, empirical, ethical, sociopolitical, spiritual, emancipatory, unknowing, aesthetic—inform understanding of caring in this nursing situation (Carper, 1978; Kagen, Smith, Cowling, & Chinn, 2009; Munhall, 1993; White, 1995)?

Personal knowing: What do I know about sickle cell disease and sickle cell crisis? What can I learn from Ms. Sands about comforting persons experiencing sickle cell crisis? What have I conveyed as a caring person? How can I be helpful to Ms. Sands and how can I be helpful to others?

Empirical knowing: What knowledge is needed to provide nursing care for a person experiencing sickle cell crisis? What knowledge is needed to understand pain? What are the genetic factors of sickle cell disease? What ongoing nursing assessments are needed? What changes are important to document and convey to all the members of the emergency room team? What do I know about supporting Ms. Sands? What patient teaching is needed for a person experiencing sickle cell crisis? What knowledge of best practice is needed to prevent complications? How does empathy sustain persons during difficult situations?

Ethical knowing: What ethical issues are present in this nursing situation? How does the code of ethics guide practice? How do Health Insurance Portability and Accountability Act (HIPAA) regulations inform nursing practice in the emergency room?

Sociopolitical knowing: What is the sociological impact of sickle cell disease? What is the impact of social stigma on care-seeking behaviors for individuals with sickle cell disease? How can the nurse support Ms. Sands and her sister to navigate the health insurance coverage for this hospital visit and treatments? How does culture impact Ms. Sands's understanding of health and sickle cell disease? What are the sociopolitical factors impacting research funding for sickle cell disease?

Spiritual knowing: How can the nurse understand the spiritual beliefs and practices of Ms. Sands? How can the nurse support Ms. Sands's spiritual needs?

Emancipatory knowing: What will it be like for Ms. Sands to live with sickle cell disease? What bureaucratic barriers may influence her recovery?

Unknowing: What matters most to Ms. Sands at this moment? How was the nurse open to understanding the nursing situation from the perspective of Ms. Sands? What did the nurse communicate through her words and actions?

Aesthetic knowing: How did the nurse support Ms. Sands's hopes and dreams? What is the beauty of this nursing situation?

What Are the Calls for Nursing?

The nurse identified empathy as the call she heard from Ms. Sands. What are some possible variations in understanding the call?

What Are the Responses to the Calls for Nursing Present in the Situation?

The nurse responded by staying with Ms. Sands, offering reassurance through her presence, calling her sister, and managing her pain with medications and complementary therapies. How did the nurse respond with authentic presence? How did the nurse respond with empathy? What nursing responses are effective in decreasing stigma for individuals with sickle cell disease?

What Was the Outcome of the Response(s) in Relation to the Call(s)?

The nurse used the philosophical perspective of caring (FAU, CON, 2012), which focuses on nurturing the wholeness and well-being of persons in caring relationships. In what way did the outcomes reflect this theoretical lens?

For the person nursed, Ms. Sands: What mattered most to Ms. Sands was for someone to stay with her and to relieve her pain.

For the nurse: The nurse learned the value of authentic presence and empathy.

For the nursing profession: This nursing situation offers an opportunity for nurses to reflect upon persons who may be stigmatized and the impact on their health and well-being.

For others: What is the value of being cared for? This nursing situation highlights the importance of nurses bearing witness to the pain and suffering of persons with chronic illness requiring frequent emergency room visits and pain management.

How Did the Study of This Nursing Situation Enhance Your Knowledge of Nursing?

What did I learn about myself as I studied this situation? What did I learn about caring science? What new possibilities can be created from this nursing situation?

LEARNING ACTIVITIES

Journal: Reflect on what happened between the nurse and one nursed.

BOX 7.1   Reflective Journal

What are your thoughts on caring expressed by the nurse in this situation?

The poem in Box 7.2 represents the nursing situation.

BOX 7.2   Aesthetic Re-presentation by the Nurse

This poem by Shirley Gordon is an aesthetic re-presentation of the nursing situation.

Knowing

Reaching out and grasping hands

Knowing eyes meeting

Touching—Connecting—Caring

Aesthetic project: How can this nursing situation be aesthetically re-presented?

BOX 7.3   Aesthetic Re-presentation

How would you aesthetically re-present this nursing situation?

REFERENCES

Carper, B. (1978). Fundamental patterns of knowing. *Advances in Nursing Science, 1*(1), 13–24.

Florida Atlantic University, Christine E. Lynn College of Nursing. (2012). *Philosophy.* Retrieved from http://nursing.fau.edu/index.php?main=1&nav=635

Kagen, P. N., Smith, M. C., Cowling, R., & Chinn, P. (2009). A nursing manifesto: An emancipatory call for nursing knowledge development, conscience, and practice. *Nursing Philosophy, 11,* 67–84.

Munhall, P. (1993). Unknowing: Toward another pattern of knowing. *Nursing Outlook, 41,* 125–128.

White, J. (1995). Patterns of knowing: Review, critique, and update. *Advances in Nursing Science, 17*(4), 73–86.

LEARNING RESOURCES

Jenerette, C. M., Lloyd, A. B., Edwards, J., Mishel, M. H., & Gil, K. M. (2014). An intervention to decrease stigma in young adults with sickle cell disease. *Western Journal of Nursing Research, 36*(5), 599–619. doi:10.1177/0193945913512724

López-Pérez, B., Ambrona, T., Gregory, J., Stocks, E., & Oceja, L. (2013). Feeling at hospitals: Perspective-taking empathy and personal distress among professional nurses and nursing students. *Nurse Education Today, 33*(4), 334–338. doi:10.1016/j.nedt.2013.01.010

Lovan, S. R., & Wilson, M. (2012). Comparing empathy levels in students at the beginning and end of a nursing program. *International Journal for Human Caring, 16*(3), 28–33.

Richardson, K., MacLeod, R., & Kent, B. (2012). A Steinian approach to an empathic understanding of hope among patients and clinicians in the culture of palliative care. *Journal of Advanced Nursing, 68*(3), 686–694. doi:10.1111/j.1365-2648.2011.05793.x

Telfer, P., Bahal, N., Lo, A., & Challands, J. (2014). Management of the acute painful crisis in sickle cell disease: A re-evaluation of the use of opioids in adult patients. *British Journal of Hematology, 166*(2), 157–164.

CHAPTER 8

Caring Between a Nurse and a Young Woman Who Experienced Sudden Cardiac Arrest in an ICU

This chapter presents a nursing situation focused on caring for Kathleen, a young woman who experienced a sudden cardiac arrest while walking along the beach. Using the philosophical perspective of caring (FAU, CON, 2012), which focuses on nurturing the wholeness and well-being of persons in caring relationships, the nursing situation highlights response to a call for nursing to provide authentic presence and empathy.

Directions: As you prepare to intentionally enter the world of the other, reflect on the following question: What are the expressions of caring between nurse and the one nursed?

NURSING SITUATION

Written by Valarie Grumme, MSN, RN, CCRN

HOPE

One of my most memorable nursing experiences involved Kathleen, a young woman who collapsed on the boardwalk in full cardiac arrest. Luckily, bystanders started chest compressions and 911 emergency responders arrived quickly. She was resuscitated and brought to our emergency room. However, she remained comatose, and paramedics were unsure of how long she was without oxygen before cardiopulmonary resuscitation (CPR) commenced. She was one of our first patients in which we initiated the new evidence-based hypothermia after cardiac arrest protocol. The goal of this therapy is to preserve brain function so the patient will awaken with no or minimal neurological deficits. The nursing staff was rooting for her.

Kathleen's fiancé (Bernard) and her parents arrived shortly after she was admitted to the unit. They were in shock—Kathleen was a healthy woman in her 20s with no known medical history. Her mother's first remark as she sobbed was, "Can't we cover her? She feels so cold." Her fiancé just stood at the bedside with tears rolling down his cheeks, and her father bent over to kiss her and let her know he was there. It was an extremely emotional situation. The next 48 hours were going to be excruciating for this family. Just as Kathleen required intense physiological monitoring, her family required intense emotional support. I asked them to tell me about Kathleen, her hopes and dreams. I encouraged the family to bring in pictures of her so that we could all see her as she lived her life. Her mom told us that Kathleen was so excited about her wedding, which was just short of 3 months away. Her friends were already planning her bridal shower.

By the next morning, her room was full of pictures. Her family continued their vigilance at her bedside. When the paralytics were discontinued, she took breaths on her own, and started moving her extremities. Her parents touched and spoke to her, and Bernard brought in her iPod so that she could hear her favorite music. You could almost feel the sense of anticipation in the room. We continued to support the family during this watchful waiting. Spiritual support from the family priest was also provided. Four hours after all sedation was stopped, Kathleen opened her eyes and followed simple commands. Everyone had tears in their eyes. She was weaned off the ventilator later that day and found to have no neurological deficits.

It was a wonderful success story. Kathleen received a full cardiovascular workup and was found to have an undiagnosed conduction disorder for which she received treatment before discharge. The nurses were invited to her wedding, and I can tell you it was a very emotional day. Kathleen and Bernard have sent us a Christmas card every year since this happened, and 2 years ago the card showed a beautiful picture of them with their new daughter. They continue to thank us for our caring, encouragement, and unwavering support. The essence of caring in this nursing situation is hope.

Within the nursing situation, the life experiences of the patient and family contribute to their vision of hope and all of its possibilities. Helping to care for this patient and her family prompted me to take a more active role in hope-facilitation as a caring practice through listening and immersing myself within each situation. An open-ended question—Tell me what your hopes are for today—is now part of my patient and family rounds.

STUDY PROCESSES

The Barry, Gordon & King Teaching/Learning Nursing Framework process is a broad guide to study and analyze nursing situations, focusing on the caring between the nurse and one nursed. In caring for this person and her family, the nurse reaches out from inside the core of the nursing situation to the periphery to explore particular caring concepts that bring the situation to life; to find relevant characteristics of the person, nurse, and environment unique to the situation; and to examine the knowledge needed to care for this person and her family. The following analysis guides and inspires understanding of nursing from the philosophical perspective of caring (FAU, CON, 2012), focusing on nurturing the wholeness and well-being of persons in caring relationships.

What Was the Caring Between the Nurse and the One Nursed?

The nurse was authentically present and provided competent, compassionate, and respectful care for Kathleen and her family as she underwent a hypothermia medical intervention designed to preserve brain function. What caring concepts opened the door for that which mattered most in the moment for this person and her family? What caring components from Roach (1987/2002) (competence, compassion, confidence, commitment, conscience, or comportment), or Mayeroff's (1971) caring ingredients (knowing, patience, alternating rhythms, humility, hope, trust, honesty, or courage) are the most important in this situation? What other expressions of caring, such as authentic presence, silence, or listening, were helpful here?

Using the Ways of Knowing, How Can We Come to Understand the Call(s) for Nursing?

How does each of the ways of knowing—personal, empirical, ethical, sociopolitical, spiritual, emancipatory, unknowing, aesthetic—inform understanding of caring in this nursing situation (Carper, 1978; Kagen, Smith, Cowling, & Chinn, 2009; Munhall, 1993; White, 1995)?

Personal knowing: What do I need to know about myself and this person and her family to care for them? Who am I as a caring person? How am I living caring as a professional nurse? Who is this person as caring fiancé and daughter? How are this person, her fiancé, and her family living caring? What personal knowledge do I bring to this situation? Do I know other relatives and friends who have experienced this health situation? Have I ever cared for a person and family with this health situation before? What did I learn from that experience? How does that influence my caring in this unique situation?

Empirical knowing: What does the nurse need to know to be technologically competent to care for a person receiving hypothermia protocol? What evidence-based research guides caring for Kathleen? What knowledge from other disciplines can inform understanding of Kathleen's unique situation? What treatments will be necessary to sustain her being until she is slowly taken out of her induced coma? What complementary modalities could be helpful for her family? What additional caring interventions could be done for her fiancé and family?

Ethical knowing: How should the nurse care for Kathleen and her family? How do the values of the theoretical perspective guide the nursing care for Kathleen and her family? How do professional ethical codes for nurses guide caring for Kathleen and her family? Is the nurse trustworthy and honest with her family? Is the nurse keeping her personal information confidential?

Sociopolitical knowing: What is the context of Kathleen's life? Who are her family members? What environmental factors may have influenced her well-being? What local, state, and federal policies and laws are impacting her well-being? What social structures impact the practice of nursing in this situation?

Spiritual knowing: How should the nurse support Kathleen and her family's religious and/or spiritual beliefs and practices? What rituals are important to her and her family?

Emancipatory knowing: How can the nurse respond to any injustices Kathleen's family might feel about her care? What are the injustices or power struggles between the family and the health care team? What advocacy is needed, and how can the nurse advocate for Kathleen?

Unknowing: How should the nurse come to understand the one nursed? How can the nurse bracket what she knows about the individual from the chart and report, while she comes to know the one nursed as a person uniquely living caring in this situation? What is learned about the individual from this unknowing effort? What are the individual's thoughts and feelings about this situation? What matters most to him or her at this time?

Aesthetic knowing: How can the nurse support Kathleen's hopes and dreams? How can the nurse transcend this moment to create possibilities? What metaphors or artistic expressions could represent the caring between the nurse and Kathleen and her family? How does the nurse weave what she has learned from all ways of knowing into the fabric of caring for Kathleen?

What Are the Calls for Nursing?

The nurse identified the essence of caring in this nursing situation as hope. Through her authentic presence she heard the call to understand their fear, sadness, and hope for Kathleen's survival.

What Are the Responses to the Calls for Nursing Present in the Situation?

The nurse responded with compassion, competence, and making every moment alive with possibilities, which inspired hope for recovery for Kathleen and her family.

What Was the Outcome of the Response in Relation to the Call(s)?

The nurse used the philosophical perspective of caring (FAU, CON, 2012), which focuses on nurturing the wholeness and well-being of persons in caring relationships. In what way did the outcomes reflect this theoretical lens?

For the person nursed, Kathleen: What mattered most to Kathleen was to survive and to become the bride she had been dreaming of. She invited all the nurses to her wedding to share in her happiness and lived out hopes and dreams.

For the nurse: Helping to care for Kathleen and her family prompted the nurse to take a more active role in hope-facilitation as a caring practice through listening and immersing herself within each situation. An open-ended question—Tell me what your hopes are for today?—is now part of her patient and family rounds.

For the nursing profession: This nursing situation exemplifies the nurse's intention to focus on the one nursed within the context of receiving the hypo-thermia post-cardiac arrest protocol demonstrating the synergistic value of technology and caring in nursing.

For others: What is the value of being cared for? This nursing situation highlights the value of caring as demonstrated by Kathleen's wedding that took place 3 months after her cardiac arrest and the rippling effect of her presence in the world.

How Did the Study of This Nursing Situation Enhance Your Knowledge of Nursing?

What did I learn about myself as I studied this situation? What did I learn about caring science? What new possibilities can be created from this nursing situation?

LEARNING ACTIVITIES

Journal: Reflect on the courage needed by the nurse bearing witness to the pain and suffering of persons.

BOX 8.1   Reflective Journal

What are your thoughts on caring expressed by the nurse in this situation?

Aesthetic re-presentation: The nurse represents the beauty of this nursing situation in the description and painting.

BOX 8.2   Aesthetic Re-presentation by the Nurse

This is Valarie Grumme's aesthetic re-presentation of her nursing situation.

Hope is a kaleidoscopic concept expressed in many shapes and forms. Facilitating hope is a key component of holistic nursing practice. My nursing situation related a memorable lived experience of helping to care for Kathleen, a young woman who survived a cardiac arrest after being placed on our hypothermia protocol. All of our care for Kathleen and her family was focused on supporting the hope that Kathleen would survive and awaken without neurological deficit. Kathleen was due to be married in less than 3 months. Her life was focused on the wedding and the start of a new family. While researching the concept of hope, my thoughts focused on Kathleen's story, and I visualized a hope chest to express the key attributes of hope identified in this situation: anticipation, spirituality, perseverance, and personal meaning. My aesthetic rendition of hope via watercolor expresses my interpretation and understanding of this complex concept.

The hope chest with its carved rainbow represents Kathleen's hopes and dreams. In the chest are items reflecting anticipation (the ring-bearer pillow, wedding garter, wedding picture frame), spirituality (the rosary), and personal meaning (a special afghan, music, and teddy bear). The "Our 1st Christmas" ornament represents perseverance, her will to survive and live life as a new family. The growing plant signifies that hope is alive. The window represents looking to the future. The frame is also special; it represents hope and all of its endless possibilities.

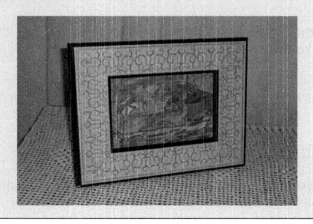

BOX 8.3   Aesthetic Re-presentation

How would you aesthetically re-present this nursing situation?

REFERENCES

Carper, B. (1978). Fundamental patterns of knowing. *Advances in Nursing Science, 1*(1), 13–24.

Florida Atlantic University, Christine E. Lynn College of Nursing. (2012). *Philosophy.* Retrieved from http://nursing.fau.edu/index.php?main=1&nav=635

Kagen, P. N., Smith, M. C., Cowling, R., & Chinn, P. (2009). A nursing manifesto: An emancipatory call for nursing knowledge development, conscience, and practice. *Nursing Philosophy, 11*, 67–84.

Mayeroff, M. (1971). *On caring.* New York, NY: HarperCollins.

Munhall, P. (1993). Unknowing: Toward another pattern of knowing. *Nursing Outlook, 41*, 125–128.

Roach, M. S. (1987/2002). *Caring, the human mode of being: A blueprint for the health professions (2nd rev. ed.).* Ottawa, Canada: The Canadian Hospital Association Press.

White, J. (1995). Patterns of knowing: Review, critique, and update. *Advances in Nursing Science, 17*(4), 73–86.

LEARNING RESOURCES

Bremer, A., Dahlberg, K., & Sandman, L. (2009). To survive out-of-hospital cardiac arrest: A search for meaning and coherence. *Qualitative Health Research, 19*(3), 323–338. doi:10.1177/1049732309331866

Froslund, A. S., Zingmark, K., Jansson, J. H., Lundblad, D., & Soderberg, S. (2014). Meanings of people's lived experiences of surviving an out-of-hospital cardiac arrest, 1 month after the event. *Journal of Cardiovascular Nursing, 29*(5), 464–471. doi:10.1097/JCN.0b013e3182a08aed

Haywood, K. L., Whitehead, L., & Perkins, G. D. (2014). The psychosocial outcomes of cardiac arrest: Relevant and robust patient-centered assessment is essential. *Resuscitation, 85*(6), 718–719. doi:10.1016/Resuscitation.2014.03.305

Ketilsdottir, A., Albertsdottir, H. R., Akadottir, S. H., Gunnarsdottir, T. J., & Jonsdottir, H. (2014). The experience of sudden cardiac arrest: Becoming reawakened to life. *European Journal of Cardiovascular Nursing, 13*(5), 429–435. doi:10.1177/1474515113504864

Larsson, I. M. (2014). *Post-cardiac arrest care: Therapeutic hypothermia, patient outcomes and relatives' experiences* (Unpublished doctoral dissertation). Uppsala University, Sweden.

McKean, S. (2009). Induced moderate hypothermia after cardiac arrest. *AACN Advanced Critical Care, 20*(4), 342–353. doi:10.1097/NCI.0b013e3181bcea4e

Nelms, T. P., & Eggenberger, S. K. (2010). The essence of the family critical illness experience and nurse-family meetings. *Journal of Family Nursing, 16*(4), 462–486. doi:10.1177/1074840710386608

Neumar, R., Otto, C., Link, M., Kronick, S., Shuster, M., Callaway, C., . . . Morrison, L. (2010). Part 8: Adult advanced cardiovascular life support 2010 American Heart Association guidelines for cardiopulmonary resuscitation and emergency cardiovascular care. *Circulation, 122*(suppl. 3), S729–S767. doi:10.1161/CIRCULATIONAHA.110.970988

Parnia, S., Spearpoint, K., & Fenwick, P. B. (2007). Near death experiences, cognitive function and psychological outcomes of surviving cardiac arrest. *Resuscitation, 74*, 215–221. doi:10.1016/j.resuscitation.2007.01.020

Parnia, S., Spearpoint, K., de Vos, G., Fenwick, P., Goldberg, D., Yang, J., & Schoenfeld, E. R. (2014). AWARE—AWAreness during REsuscitation—A prospective study. *Resuscitation, 85*(12), 1799–1805. doi:10.1016/j.resuscitation.2014.09.004

Wallin, E., Larsson, I. M., Rubertsson, S., & Kristoferzon, M. L. (2013). Relatives' experiences of everyday life six months after hypothermia treatment of a significant other's cardiac arrest. *Journal of Clinical Nursing, 22*(11–12), 1639–1644. doi:10.1111/jocn.12112

CHAPTER 9

Caring Between a Nurse and an Adult in an ICU Setting

This chapter presents a nursing situation focused on caring for an adult woman in the intensive care unit (ICU), suffering with pneumonia following a cholecystectomy. Using the philosophical perspective of caring (FAU, CON, 2012), which focuses on nurturing the wholeness and well-being of persons in caring relationships, the nursing situation highlights the person's courage as she faces the unknown.

Directions: As you prepare to intentionally enter the world of the other, reflect on the following question: What are the expressions of caring between the nurse and the one nursed?

NURSING SITUATION

Written by Dana Reynolds, BSN, RN

ENGAGING EYES

Mrs. Gonzales, a 46-year-old female, was admitted to my care experiencing nausea, vomiting, abdominal pain, and a fever of 101°F. Mrs. Gonzales was quickly diagnosed with cholecystitis and later developed tachypnea and respiratory distress. Her oxygen saturation was 88% on nasal cannula at 2L. A chest x-ray revealed a diagnosis of pneumonia. I reassured her as she was being transferred to the operating room.

My next encounter with Mrs. Gonzales was following surgery. She was intubated during surgery and continued on PRVC ventilator support. She had received Propofol but, surprisingly, was awake and alert. Mrs. Gonzales was able to follow simple commands and nod appropriately when questioned about pain. When she saw me, I noticed right away that she recognized me, as her eyes demonstrated relief. If she had not been intubated, I think she would have said, "Finally! Where have you been?" I stroked her head gently, and stated, "Do not worry, Mrs. Gonzales. I am here." She nodded her head in understanding.

Mrs. Gonzales remained intubated over the next 10 days and experienced several unsuccessful extubation attempts that required immediate re-intubation. It became evident that Mrs. Gonzales was growing restless, depressed, and anxious whenever she was informed of a failed extubation trial. I had developed a fondness for her and wanted her to succeed in her extubation attempts.

Her chest x-ray and arterial blood gases (ABGs) had greatly improved and she was ready for the tube to be removed. After discussions of possible tracheostomy placement if weaning was unsuccessful, I was determined to help her get extubated successfully. I consulted and devised a plan with the intensivist for a scheduled time for morning "sedation vacation"— medication to be given for anxiety, and meds for pain. After receiving her med cocktail and turning off her Propofol, Mrs. Gonzales's vent settings were changed to continuous positive airway pressure (CPAP). I held her hand and told her, "This is it. We are going to get this out today, right?" Mrs. Gonzales nodded her head in agreement. In order to keep her calm, I combed and washed her hair, stroked her arm gently, and watched her favorite telenovela with her (even though I did not understand Spanish).

Every so often Mrs. Gonzales would glance over at me with such sincerity and appreciation. Two hours went by without sedation, no anxiety, and no tachypnea. She was ready. Before extubation, I looked at Mrs. Gonzales and said, "This is it; this is what we have been waiting for. You can do it, just remember to breathe." She practiced her breathing and in a matter of seconds, with engaging eyes between the two of us, she was extubated!

Her vitals remained stable, and she exhibited no tachypnea post-extubation. Although she was instructed not to speak, she looked at me with her big bright eyes and whispered, "Thank you!" I was elated for her, proud at what we accomplished together. I kissed her on the forehead and replied, "I told you we could do it!" Later that day she told her son that she loved me and appreciated everything I did for her. All I could say was, "I love you, too." The essence of caring in this nursing situation is love.

STUDY PROCESSES

The Barry, Gordon & King Teaching/Learning Nursing Framework process is a broad guide to study and analyze nursing situations, focusing on the caring between the nurse and one nursed. In caring for Mrs. Gonzales, the nurse was determined to help her become extubated. Using her nursing knowledge, authentic presence, and independent nursing responses, she assisted Mrs. Gonzales to be successfully weaned from the respirator. The following analysis guides and inspires understanding of nursing from the philosophical perspective of caring (FAU, CON, 2012), focusing on nurturing the wholeness and well-being of persons in caring relationships.

What Was the Caring Between the Nurse and the One Nursed?

The nurse identified love as the essence of caring. Expressions of caring between the nurse and Mrs. Gonzales included trust, respect, hope, and dignity. What caring behaviors by the nurse were present? How did the nurse instill trust with Mrs. Gonzales? How did the nurse assist Mrs. Gonzales with maintaining hope with each unsuccessful extubation attempt? What other caring concepts by Roach (2002) or caring ingredients by Mayeroff (1971) are present in this nursing situation?

Using the Ways of Knowing, How Can We Come to Understand the Call(s) for Nursing?

How does each of the ways of knowing—personal, empirical, ethical, sociopolitical, spiritual, emancipatory, unknowing, aesthetic—inform understanding of caring in this nursing situation (Carper, 1978; Kagen, Smith, Cowling, & Chinn, 2009; Munhall, 1993; White, 1995)?

Personal knowing: How can I understand the fear Mrs. Gonzales must be experiencing? What do I know about how to support a person during extubation? What do I know about the Hispanic culture? How can I help her when I do not speak her language? How am I living caring? What personal knowledge do I have of this situation?

Empirical knowing: What knowledge is needed to understand the disease processes of pneumonia and cholecystitis? What knowledge is needed about her medications, such as Propofol? What does the oxygen level of 88% signify? What are the normal values for ABGs? What knowledge of evidence-based practice is needed to care for a person on a ventilator? What are the signs of infection post-operation? What nursing responses might be appropriate to decrease Mrs. Gonzales's anxiety?

Ethical knowing: What ethical issues are present in this situation? Is the nurse honest and truthful with Mrs. Gonzales? How do codes of ethics guide practice?

Sociopolitical knowing: What is the context of Mrs. Gonzales' life, home, family, work, and friends, and how might these influence recovery? What is the relationship between economic status and health outcomes? How do cultural beliefs impact Mrs. Gonzales's understanding?

Spiritual knowing: How can the nurse help sustain Mrs. Gonzales's sense of hope? How can the nurse support Mrs. Gonzales's spiritual beliefs and practices?

Emancipatory knowing: How can the nurse advocate for Mrs. Gonzales? In a hierarchical system, how can nurses make their voices heard?

Unknowing: What does the nurse not know about Mrs. Gonzales? How is the nurse open to what Mrs. Gonzales is communicating? How can the nurse come to understand Mrs. Gonzales's needs, hopes, and dreams?

Aesthetic knowing: What is the beauty of the moment when Mrs. Gonzales breathes on her own? How can the nurse express her love and care for Mrs. Gonzales?

What Are the Calls for Nursing?

The nurse hears the call from Mrs. Gonzales to help her breathe on her own, to stay with her, and to keep her safe. What other calls for nursing are present in this nursing situation? How do the ways of knowing inform understanding of the calls? How does the nurse prioritize the numerous calls of Mrs. Gonzales?

What Are the Responses to the Calls for Nursing Present in the Situation?

The nurse responded with competence and vigilance in assisting Mrs. Gonzales to breathe on her own. How did the nurse express caring? What are other possible responses to the calls for nursing?

What Was the Outcome of the Response?

The nurse used the philosophical perspective of caring (FAU, CON, 2012), which focuses on nurturing the wholeness and well-being of persons in caring relationships.

In what way did the outcomes reflect this theoretical lens?

For the person nursed, Mrs. Gonzales: What mattered most to Mrs. Gonzales was to breathe on her own, recover from surgery, and return home.

For the nurse: The nurse learned the value of the interprofessional team working in collaboration with Mrs. Gonzales toward the outcomes for which they hoped.

For the nursing profession: The value of caring, interprofessional collaboration, and advocacy are essential to cost-effective care and enhanced health outcomes.

For others: What is the value of being cared for? What impact does inter-professional collaboration have on the economics of health care?

How Did the Study of This Nursing Situation Enhance Your Knowledge of Nursing?

What did I learn about nursing in this situation? What did I learn about caring science? What new possibilities can be created from this nursing situation?

LEARNING ACTIVITIES

Journal: Reflect on what happened between Mrs. Gonzales and the nurse.

BOX 9.1   Reflective Journal

What are your thoughts on caring expressed by the nurse in this situation?

Re-presentation aesthetic project: The poem in Box 9.2 represents the nursing situation.

BOX 9.2   Aesthetic Re-presentation by the Nurse

This is Dana Reynolds's aesthetic re-presentation of her nursing situation.

The nurse re-presented the nursing situation via poetry. She indicated her poem signified love in a silent moment between the patient and nurse. The poem was displayed with a gold frame, which exemplified strength and love in its powerful union of words. In her practice, the nurse expressed that it was important to build a strong foundation with patients. That foundation was grounded in trust, advocacy, and empathy. She states, "I feel like if the foundation is not real, or forced, the patient does not benefit in obtaining the best possible care. Love is the answer."

"Silent Conversation of Love"
Awake, alert, and intubated
Silence between us but a mutual love, and respect is felt in the air.
Her eyes close gently as I stroke her hair.
Appreciation.
As much as you yearn for this giant tube to be taken from your throat, so do I.
Understanding.
As we prepare for extubation you hold my hand gently, as I whisper in your ear
"It's ok Ada, Just breathe."
Freedom.
Although you are told not to speak, you look at me and say "Thank You!"
A kiss on the forehead to seal the deal.
Love.

Aesthetic project: How can this nursing situation be aesthetically re-presented?

BOX 9.3   Aesthetic Re-presentation

How would you aesthetically re-present this nursing situation?

REFERENCES

Carper, B. (1978). Fundamental patterns of knowing. *Advances in Nursing Science, 1*(1), 13–24.

Florida Atlantic University, Christine E. Lynn College of Nursing. (2012). *Philosophy.* Retrieved from http://nursing.fau.edu/index.php?main=1&nav=635

Kagen, P. N., Smith, M. C., Cowling, R., & Chinn, P. (2009). A nursing manifesto: An emancipatory call for nursing knowledge development, conscience, and practice. *Nursing Philosophy, 11,* 67–84.

Mayeroff, M. (1971). *On caring.* New York, NY: Harper Perennial.

Munhall, P. (1993). Unknowing: Toward another pattern of knowing. *Nursing Outlook, 41,* 125–128.

Roach, S. (2002). *Caring, the human mode of being* (2nd ed.). Ottawa, Canada: Canadian Health Association.

White, J. (1995). Patterns of knowing: Review, critique, and update. *Advances in Nursing Science, 17*(4), 73–86.

LEARNING RESOURCES

American Association of Critical-Care Nurses (AACN; 2008). Practice Alerts. *Ventilator associated pneumonia.* Retrieved from http://www.aacn.org/WD/Practice/Docs/Ventilator_Associated_Pneumonia_1-2008.pdf

Centers for Disease Control and Prevention. (2015a). *Healthcare associated infections.* Retrieved from http://www.cdc.gov/hai/vap/vap.html

Centers for Disease Control and Prevention. (2015b). *National healthcare safety network.* Retrieved from http://www.cdc.gov/nhsn/acute-care-hospital/vap/

Leininger, M., & McFarland, M. (2006). *Culture care diversity and universality: A worldwide nursing theory.* Boston, MA: Jones & Bartlett.

Ray, M. (2009). *Transcultural caring dynamics in nursing and healthcare.* Philadelphia, PA: F.A. Davis.

U.S. Department of Health and Human Services/Office of Minority Health. (2015). Retrieved from http://minorityhealth.hhs.gov/

U.S. Department of Health and Human Services, Office of Minority Health. (2001). *National standards for culturally and linguistically appropriate health services in health care: Executive summary.* Washington, DC: Author.

CHAPTER 10

Caring Between a Nurse and a Young Adult Experiencing Cancer

This chapter presents a nursing situation focused on caring for a young woman with uterine cancer. Using the philosophical perspective of caring (FAU, CON, 2012), which focuses on nurturing the wholeness and well-being of persons in caring relationships, the nursing situation highlights the courage of both the nurse and one nursed.

Directions: As you prepare to intentionally enter the world of the other, reflect on the following question: What are the expressions of caring between nurse and the one nursed?

NURSING SITUATION

Written by Margarita Dorsey, BSN, RN, CCRN

THE QUEEN AND HER FAMILY

Mrs. Quinn, a person I cared for before my ICU days, has never left my heart. She was a 30-year-old woman hospitalized in a step down unit. Immediately I pegged her for an easy admit and discharge. The other nurses avoided her room, and I figured it was because she was ornery and staff was not able to deal with her. I was assigned to her because I was the only one that did not refuse. Armed with this false sense of who she was and half expecting a demanding rude patient, I started my shift and opened her door. I was taken aback by how beautiful she was. She was a fit, young woman from the Caribbean, with gorgeous tan skin and a little black pixie haircut. Her sweet young children, a boy and a girl, were lying beside her. Her husband was at her bedside, despondent with his head in her lap as she stroked his hair. She looked like a queen consoling her king. Her big doe eyes met mine, and if I could say there were a moment God Almighty Himself put me right where I needed to be, it was at that moment. She had stage four uterine cancer with metastasis to the lungs and bone. I couldn't wrap my mind around how somebody who looked better than I did physically could be so sick. I proceeded to care for her, took her vital signs, and offered her medication as ordered. When asked how she was feeling, she barely spoke to me.

When her family left the following morning, her stoic guard collapsed. She waited until her husband and children left before she let her true feelings show. She told me her story, how quickly she was diagnosed, and stated, "As a woman and mother, I have to be strong for them. Do you mind if I cry with you?" It was time for my shift to end, and I ended up spending 3 hours after my shift just talking to her, listening, consoling, and being present in the moment. She said I reminded her of her sister. She explained how she accepted God's challenge but lived in the real fear of leaving her family behind. There was a solid strength in her that awed me and as we spoke like two old friends, I felt Godly agape love. Her realness with me was baffling. I could see she bottled up all these emotions for the sake of her family and I was happy to be her shoulder to cry on. She told me something that will resonate with me forever: "I may not ever know for sure why I was put on this earth, but I sure hope that I left the people I loved in life in a better state than I found them. I won't question God, because His will is sovereign over anything, but I'm a human. I'm scared and I'm not ashamed of that."

I washed her hair and massaged her feet before I left, and we shared a final hug. I was so devastated that something so bad was happening to somebody so nice that I admit that I questioned Almighty God as to why these terrible diagnoses plague people. I understand why colleagues refused her as a patient now. It physically hurt me to take care of her, because I cared about her so much. The essence of caring in this nursing situation is courage.

STUDY PROCESSES

The Barry, Gordon & King Teaching/Learning Nursing Framework process is a broad guide to study and analyze nursing situations, focusing on the caring between the nurse and one nursed. The following analysis guides and inspires understanding of nursing from the philosophical perspective of caring (FAU, CON, 2012), focusing on nurturing the wholeness and well-being of persons in caring relationships.

What Was the Caring Between the Nurse and the One Nursed?

The nurse states, "It takes courage to care for patients who are actively suffering." The nursing staff was reluctant to care for Mrs. Quinn because many of them saw themselves in her—a mother and wife who wanted to live for her family. It took a tremendous amount of courage for the nurse to enter Mrs. Quinn's world and witness her fears and trials. Mrs. Quinn turned to the nurse for support. What other caring concepts are expressed in this nursing situation?

Using the Ways of Knowing, How Can We Come to Understand the Call(s) for Nursing?

How does each of the ways of knowing—personal, empirical, ethical, sociopolitical, spiritual, emancipatory, unknowing, aesthetic—inform understanding of caring in this nursing situation (Carper, 1978; Kagen, Smith, Cowling, & Chinn, 2009; Munhall, 1993; White, 1995)?

Personal knowing: Who am I as a caring person? Who is Mrs. Quinn as a caring person? What personal knowing do I bring to this situation? What do I know about caring for a person with terminal cancer? What are my own spiritual beliefs related to health, illness, and death?

Empirical knowing: What knowledge is needed to care for a person with Stage 4 uterine cancer? What knowledge of death and dying is needed to care for Mrs. Quinn? What are the evidence-based practices for pain management? In addition to foot massage, what complementary modalities could be helpful in caring for Mrs. Quinn? What knowledge is needed to care for Mrs. Quinn's family? What therapeutic communication techniques would be beneficial to enhancing the well-being of Mrs. Quinn?

Ethical knowing: What ethical principles are present in this nursing situation? How do the codes of ethics guide practice? How did the nurse fulfill professional obligations to Mrs. Quinn? How would advance directives influence nursing care for Mrs. Quinn?

Sociopolitical knowing: How do Mrs. Quinn's cultural beliefs impact her health and well-being? How does Mrs. Quinn's role as wife and mother influence her understanding in decision making? What is the meaning of stoicism for Mrs. Quinn and her family? What knowledge is needed to understand how Mrs. Quinn's financial status may influence end-of-life care?

Spiritual knowing: How should I support Mrs. Quinn's religious and/or spiritual beliefs and practices?

Unknowing: What mattered most to Mrs. Quinn at this moment in time? What do we know about Mrs. Quinn from her husband and children? How could the nurse remain open to understanding Mrs. Quinn, her family, and colleagues?

Emancipatory knowing: How could the nurse advocate for Mrs. Quinn in this nursing situation? How do the laws related to citizenship and immigration impact health care? What barriers to Mrs. Quinn's care are present?

Aesthetic knowing: What was the beauty of nursing in this nursing situation? How could this nursing situation be re-presented aesthetically?

What Are the Calls for Nursing?

The nurse identifies the call for authentic presence and to listen to her hopes and fears. What other calls may be present? What mattered most to Mrs. Quinn at this moment in time? What might be "unspoken" calls? What are the calls from her family?

What Are the Responses to the Calls for Nursing Present in the Nursing Situation?

The nurse responded to the call by demonstrating courage as she listened to Mrs. Quinn's story. Massaging her feet, washing her hair, and giving her hugs and love are all responses to the human call for authentic presence. What other nursing responses could be provided? What nursing responses are needed to assist the family?

What Was the Outcome of the Response(s) in Relation to the Call(s)?

The nurse used the philosophical perspective of caring (FAU, CON, 2012), which focuses on nurturing the wholeness and well-being of persons in caring relationships. In what way did the outcomes reflect this theoretical lens?

For the person nursed, Mrs. Quinn: What mattered most to Mrs. Quinn was her children, husband, and her need to be strong in front of them.

For the nurse: The nurse learned the value of courage needed for authentic presence.

For the nursing profession: This nursing situation offers an opportunity for nurses to review their ethical obligations for persons nursed and in accepting or rejecting assignments.

For others: What is the value of being cared for? Understanding the importance of bearing witness to the pain and suffering of persons with terminal cancer is invaluable to society.

How Did the Study of This Nursing Situation Enhance Your Knowledge of Nursing?

What did I learn about myself as I studied this situation? What did I learn about caring science? What new possibilities can be created from this nursing situation?

LEARNING ACTIVITIES

Journal: Reflect on the courage needed by the nurse bearing witness to the pain and suffering of persons.

BOX 10.1   Reflective Journal

What are your thoughts on caring expressed by the nurse in this situation?

Aesthetic re-presentation: How can this nursing situation be aesthetically re-presented?

BOX 10.2   Aesthetic Re-presentation

How would you aesthetically re-present this nursing situation?

REFERENCES

Carper, B. (1978). Fundamental patterns of knowing. *Advances in Nursing Science, 1*(1), 13–24.

Florida Atlantic University, Christine E. Lynn College of Nursing. (2012). *Philosophy*. Retrieved from http://nursing.fau.edu/index.php?main=1&nav=635

Kagen, P. N., Smith, M. C., Cowling, R., & Chinn, P. (2009). A nursing manifesto: An emancipatory call for nursing knowledge development, conscience, and practice. *Nursing Philosophy, 11*, 67–84.

Munhall, P. (1993). Unknowing: Toward another pattern of knowing. *Nursing Outlook, 41*, 125–128.

White, J. (1995). Patterns of knowing: Review, critique, and update. *Advances in Nursing Science, 17*(4), 73–86.

LEARNING RESOURCES

American Psychological Association. (2015). *Death & dying*. Retrieved from http://apa.org/topics/death/index.aspx

Cowan, R. (Producer), Winkler, I. (Producer), & Winkler, I. (Director). (2001). *Life as a House* (Motion Picture). New York, NY: Winkler Films.

Field, S. (Producer), McCormick, K. (Producer), Henderson, D., & Schumacher, J. (Director). (1991). *Dying young* (Motion picture). Los Angeles, CA: Fogwood Films Twentieth Fox Film Corporation.

Hawkins, S., & Morse, J. (2014). The praxis of courage as a foundation for care. *Journal of Nursing Scholarship, 46*(4), 263–270.

National Cancer Institute at the National Institutes of Health. (2015a). *Endometrial cancer*. Retrieved from http://www.cancer.gov/cancertopics/types/endometrial

National Cancer Institute at the National Institutes of Health. (2015b). *Uterine cancer*. Retrieved from http://www.cancer.gov/cancertopics/types/uterine

CHAPTER 11

Caring Among a Nurse and a Mother, Father, and Baby in the NICU

This chapter presents a nursing situation focused on caring for a newborn baby girl, as well as her mother and father. Using the philosophical perspective of caring (FAU, CON, 2012), which focuses on nurturing the wholeness and well-being of persons in caring relationships, the nursing situation highlights the nurse's authentic presence.

Directions: As you prepare to intentionally enter the world of the other, reflect on the following question: What are the expressions of caring between nurse and the one nursed?

NURSING SITUATION

WRITTEN BY KARMEL McCARTHY-RICHES, MAOM, BSN, RN

END OF DAY END OF SHIFT

It was just another ordinary day at work. I was working in my usual assigned area of the neonatal intensive care unit. Happily ensconced with my thriving preemies, it was going to be a good day. Little did I know that by the end of the day, the end of my shift, an event would occur that would eventually change the way I practiced the art of nursing.

As the day progressed, I cared for my littlest patients and their families. Being there for the families every step of the way was something on which I prided myself. That afternoon, the NICU received a phone call from the labor and delivery unit alerting us to the fact that a patient in room seven had thick meconium and they would be expecting us to attend the delivery. As was normal practice, I went to the room in advance of the delivery to check the neonatal resuscitation equipment. Entering the room, I encountered a young couple expecting their first baby. Mrs. Mott had received an epidural and was feeling no pain. The room was full of excitement as both sets of grandparents were there awaiting the arrival of their first grandchild. I happily answered their questions, as they were naturally concerned about the baby having meconium-stained amniotic fluid. I reassured them that this was something we see all the time. When I approached Mrs. Mott to ask her if she had any questions, she was quick to say no as she had already spoken to her obstetrician about the meconium. With my equipment check done, I retreated to the NICU. I wasn't there but an hour when we received word from labor and delivery that Mrs. Mott was ready to deliver. Off I went to attend the delivery.

When I entered the room, accompanied by the neonatologist, delivery was imminent. I stood by the radiant warmer holding a blanket for the baby under the heat source so it would be warm for the baby. As Mrs. Mott continued to push, the heat bore down on my head and neck. It was the end of the shift, change of shift to be exact. I was tired. All I could think about was going home to my husband and children. I did not want to be there in that moment, but I pretended to be excited for the family. I took on the role I thought I was supposed to play in that moment. Finally, the baby arrived.

Silence. It was deafening to my trained ears. There was no initial cry. The neonatologist placed the limp, blue baby on the radiant warmer. We knew immediately something was wrong. The baby required intensive resuscitation. Finally, after 5 minutes, she cried. It was a weak and feeble cry, but she cried. At that minute, the tension-filled room filled with gasps of relief. "Is she okay? Is she okay?" Mrs. Mott asked repeatedly. I could not answer. The obstetrician kept offering reassuring words to the mother. However, the obstetrician was not seeing what we were seeing. The deformities were clear. She was small, she had rocker bottom feet, her delicate long fingers were overlapped and clenched, her heart sounds reverberated with a loud murmur. I still can hear that murmur if I listen quietly in my mind. Trisomy 18 is what we suspected. While the neonatologist spoke to the family, I prepared her for transport to the NICU.

I wrapped her small body in a warm soft blanket and covered her tiny head with a pink hat. All you could see was her perfect little face. She was perfect in her parents' eyes. I showed the parents their baby girl and I will never forget Mrs. Mott looking into my eyes and asking me to please take care of her baby. I reassured her I would.

In the NICU, the staff came quickly together to stabilize the baby. IV pumps beeping, cardiac monitors alarming. As the hours passed, it was clear that the baby girl was not going to survive. Mr. and Mrs. Mott were given the devastating news. Their cries shattered the silence of the unit. I stayed on past the end of my shift.

I wanted to care for this baby as promised. I wanted Mrs. Mott to know the joy of holding her baby alive; to feel the warmth of the baby next to her skin. I took the baby to her parents. I held her swaddled body close to me and sat on the side of Mrs. Mott's bed. She did not reach out for her. Tears rolled down her cheeks. She was so afraid to touch her baby girl. As I held the baby, I placed my hand gently on Mrs. Mott's leg. The hospital blanket was cold and rough to touch.

In that moment, Mrs. Mott reached out for her baby. I placed the baby in her arms. I did not leave. I sat there with my hand on her leg and I cried. I still remember the salty taste of my tears. I did not worry if this was how I was supposed to act as her nurse; I was being my true self in that moment. I was there for her birth and there for her death, which are two of the most intimate moments of one's life.

I never saw Mrs. Mott again. A year later, I received a letter from her. The letter thanked me for being present for her in her darkest hour and that I may not know how the touch of my hand gave her strength and comfort. In that moment, I knew how I wanted to practice as a nurse. The essence of caring in this nursing situation is authentic presence.

STUDY PROCESSES

The Barry, Gordon & King Teaching/Learning Nursing Framework process is a broad guide to study and analyze nursing situations, focusing on the caring between the nurse and one nursed. The following analysis guides and inspires understanding of nursing from the philosophical perspective of caring (FAU, CON, 2012), focusing on nurturing the wholeness and well-being of persons in caring relationships.

What Was the Caring Between the Nurse and the One Nursed?

The nurse cared for Mr. and Mrs. Mott and their baby girl competently through her commitment to be present, authentically listening, and offering comfort through touch. What other caring ingredients are present in this situation? How did the nurse express caring? How did the nurse's competence influence the nursing situation?

Using the Ways of Knowing, How Can We Come to Understand the Call(s) for Nursing?

How does each of the ways of knowing—personal, empirical, ethical, sociopolitical, spiritual, emancipatory, unknowing, aesthetic—inform understanding of caring in this nursing situation (Carper, 1978; Kagen, Smith, Cowling, & Chinn, 2009; Munhall, 1993; White, 1995)?

Personal knowing: What have I conveyed as a caring person? What do I need to know about the loss of a newborn? How did the nurse live caring? How did the parents live caring?

Empirical knowing: What knowledge is needed to provide nursing care to a newborn that is dying? What knowledge is needed to care for newborns immediately following delivery? What knowledge is needed to care for a family who is experiencing the death of a newborn? What is the research related to Trisomy 18? What is the influence of a child's death on family dynamics? What knowledge of family theory is needed to care for Mr. and Mrs. Mott? What best practice guides nursing in this situation?

Ethical knowing: What ethical theories guide end-of-life decision making? How did the theoretical lens guide the nurse's ethical practice? What ethical principles are lived in this nursing situation? How do codes of ethics guide nursing practice?

Sociopolitical knowing: What is the context of this family's life— grandparents, conception history, home, work, culture? How has medical technology influenced health care outcomes and costs?

Spiritual knowing: How can the nurse support Mr. and Mrs. Mott's spiritual beliefs and practices? What best practice relates to care of families who have experienced the death of a newborn?

Emancipatory knowing: What bureaucratic constraints might exist in this nursing situation? What advocacy actions are needed?

Unknowing: What did the nurse unknowingly communicate to Mr. and Mrs. Mott through her words and actions? As you reflect on the nursing care of Mr. and Mrs. Mott and their baby, what are you feeling? What mattered most to this family?

Aesthetic knowing: How did the nurse support Mr. and Mrs. Mott's hopes and dreams? How might you aesthetically represent this nursing situation?

What Are the Calls for Nursing?

The nurse heard the call to be authentically present with Mr. and Mrs. Mott as they experienced the birth and death of their newborn daughter. What other calls can you identify in this nursing situation?

What Are the Responses to the Calls for Nursing Present in the Situation?

The nurse initially responded to the call with authentic presence by staying with Mrs. Mott as she held her baby girl for the first and last time. Mrs. Mott said the nurse's touch meant so much to her in her darkest hour. The nurse also cared for her baby girl as she swaddled her in a warm soft blanket and placed a pink hat on her head as she went to say hello to her parents for the first time. What other expressions of caring are present? What other responses are possible? How did the ways of knowing inform the nurse's response?

What Was the Outcome of the Response(s) in Relation to the Call(s)?

The nurse used the philosophical perspective of caring (FAU, CON, 2012), which focuses on nurturing the wholeness and well-being of persons in caring relationships.

For the one nursed, Mr. and Mrs. Mott: What mattered most to Mr. and Mrs. Mott was their newborn. To experience both life and death in a matter of hours expresses the alternating rhythms of life.

For the nurse: The nurse learned the value of being authentically present for those in her care.

For the nursing profession: This nursing situation exemplifies the uniqueness of calls and responses and the courage of the nursing profession as witnesses of pain and suffering.

For others: What is the value of being cared for? Being able to provide comfort to those suffering has great economic value. The value of being present when a person enters this world and leaves this world is priceless.

How Did the Study of This Nursing Situation Enhance Your Knowledge of Nursing?

What did I learn about myself as I studied this situation? What did I learn about caring science? What new possibilities can be created from this nursing situation?

LEARNING ACTIVITIES

Journal: Reflect on the alternating rhythms of your own life. Who has been present and cared for you?

BOX 11.1   Reflective Journal

Reflect on the alternating rhythms of your own life. Who has been present and cared for you?

Aesthetic re-presentation: How can this nursing situation be aesthetically re-presented?

BOX 11.2   Aesthetic Re-presentation

How would you aesthetically re-present this nursing situation?

REFERENCES

Carper, B. (1978). Fundamental patterns of knowing. *Advances in Nursing Science, 1*(1), 13–24.

Florida Atlantic University, Christine E. Lynn College of Nursing. (2012). *Philosophy.* Retrieved from http://nursing.fau.edu/index.php?main=1&nav=635

Kagen, P. N., Smith, M. C., Cowling, R., & Chinn, P. (2009). A nursing manifesto: An emancipatory call for nursing knowledge development, conscience, and practice. *Nursing Philosophy, 11,* 67–84.

Munhall, P. (1993). Unknowing: Toward another pattern of knowing. *Nursing Outlook, 41,* 125–128.

White, J. (1995). Patterns of knowing: Review, critique, and update. *Advances in Nursing Science, 17*(4), 73–86.

LEARNING RESOURCES

Armementrout, D. C. (2009). Living with grief following removal of infant life support: Parent's perspective. *Critical Care Nursing Clinics of North American, 21*(2), 253–265.

Bereaved Parents of the USA. (2015). *A journey together.* Retrieved from http://www.bereavedparentsusa.org/

Brooten, D., Youngblut, J. M., Seagrave, L., Caicedo, C., Hawthorne, D., Hidalgo, I., & Roche, R. (2013). Parent's perceptions of health care providers actions around child ICU death: What helped, what did not. *American Journal of Hospice & Palliative Medicine, 30*(1), 40–49.

The Compassionate Friends: Supporting Families After a Child Dies. (2015). *Providing grief support after the death of a child.* Retrieved from http://www.compassionatefriends.org/home.aspx

Youngblut, J. M., Brooten, D., Cantwell, G. P., del Moral, T., & Totapally, B. (2013). Parent health and functioning 13 months after infant or child NICU/PICU death. *Pediatrics, 132*(5), 1295–1301.

CHAPTER 12

Caring Between a Nurse and a Child in an Acute Care Oncology Setting

This chapter presents a nursing situation focused on the caring between a child and her nurse. Using the philosophical perspective of caring (FAU, CON, 2012), which focuses on nurturing the wholeness and well-being of persons in caring relationships, the nursing situation highlights the simple yet complex nature of caring for a child.

Directions: As you prepare to intentionally enter the world of the other, reflect on the following question: What are the expressions of caring between nurse and the one nursed?

NURSING SITUATION

Written by Michelle Palokas, DNP, RN-CPN

HOW I LEARNED NURSING

I was a student nurse in my last semester of school; I was nervous but energetic. I knew that pediatrics was the place for me before I even entered the doors of the hospital. The day I met Sarah, my belief was confirmed. Sarah's eyes were so full of hope the first time we met. Although she was bald and frail from chemotherapy and a bone marrow transplant, her eyes gleamed. Sarah was so weak that you could barely hear her speaking voice; but she didn't complain. She smiled anyway. Her smiles were reassurance that I'd done something right—that I'd made her happy or comfortable. And though I had several other patients during my clinical rotation, there was something special about Sarah. There was an unspoken connection. To this day, I can't explain it.

One of the first days after we'd met, Sarah called out on the call light and requested my presence. At that moment, I remember thinking, "Hmmm—I wonder, *why me?* What have I done that makes her want *me* in the room over her assigned nurse?"

After graduating, I was blessed to be offered a job on this unit where we met. Sarah was a patient there, on and off, and then very consistently for almost a year. She requested me as her nurse; I requested her as my patient. We enjoyed each other's company unlike any other nurse–patient relationship that I'd experienced before or have experienced since. And I've never laughed as hard as the Halloween she spent in the hospital. Sarah was a jokester, that one! She loved practical jokes and would do almost anything, including bribing other staff members to participate.

Sarah also loved art. The art therapist was one of her favorite people and she would anxiously watch the clock on the wall when it was an art therapy day. They painted and drew, created and molded until the art therapist insisted that she must see another patient. And her drawings and paintings were always so full of color and promise. That was her happy place. When she was creating, she forgot about the graft versus host disease that was destroying her tiny 11-year-old body.

Sarah spent 99% of her days in the hospital alone. With very little family and a mother who was battling her own demons, she became used to a quiet room and an empty visitor chair. When I would inquire about her mother or the contact she had or wanted with her, she never spoke negatively or appeared angry. She was always understanding, forgiving, and wise beyond her years. Sarah's Make-a-Wish trip was to a restaurant with her mother and siblings, then shopping for her entire family. Can't we all learn a lesson from that? She could have had any trip or toy she wanted, but she chose quality time with her family and to shower *them* with gifts.

Sarah died on a Sunday. She had been in and out of consciousness for weeks, and she knew that this time was drawing near. One of the last pictures she drew was one with angels and a glowing light; and she wanted it hung on the wall at the foot of her bed so she could see it while lying in the bed. She'd barely had strength to even scratch her nose for weeks, but that day, which just happened to be my shift, I watched her lift her arms up to the heavens so willfully and easily. Although her eyes were closed, I asked, "What do you see? What are you reaching for?" And Sarah whispered, "It's Him." The tears welled up in my eyes until I couldn't contain them any longer. With her mother there at her bedside I asked for permission to pray. We prayed together and, shortly after, that picture at the end of her bed became her reality.

As I sit and reflect about my nursing career thus far, this is one patient that continues to be at the forefront of my memory. Sarah makes my heart smile every time I think of her. There is not necessarily one day or moment in time that was more special or precious than another; it is simply our journey together, as patient and nurse, and how we helped each other learn and grow.

This patient taught me patience, forgiveness, and showed me how to love unconditionally, even when it feels undeserved. Sarah also taught me that appreciation can be felt and not just heard as a "thank you." She taught me to smile when the going gets tough and to have an attitude of gratitude. She didn't complain about her illness, despair over her family situation, or wallow in self-pity. Sarah appreciated every person that was a part of her life, no matter how big or small of an impact he or she had made.

STUDY PROCESSES

The Barry, Gordon & King Teaching/Learning Nursing Framework is a broad guide to study and analyze the nursing situation, focusing on the caring between the nurse and one nursed. In caring for Sarah, the nurse reaches out from inside the core of the nursing situation to the periphery to explore particular caring concepts that bring the situation to life; to find relevant characteristics of the person, nurse, and environment unique to the situation; and to examine the knowledge needed to care for this child. Reflecting, synthesizing, and integrating knowledge from a multidisciplinary approach informs and enlivens understanding of the other. The following analysis guides and inspires understanding of nursing from the philosophical perspective of caring (FAU, CON, 2012), focusing on nurturing the wholeness and well-being of persons in caring relationships.

What Was the Caring Between the Nurse and the One Nursed?

The nurse describes the reciprocal relationship between Sarah and herself that started to build immediately upon meeting each other. She states she doesn't know why this happened and adds how they helped each other grow. She goes on to describe all the things Sarah taught her about being a nurse—patience, forgiveness, unconditional love, appreciation, gratitude, and to smile when the going gets tough.

What caring concepts opened the door for that which mattered most in the moment for this child? Was it the intention to nurse from a particular theory of caring science? What caring components from Roach (1987/2002)—competence, compassion, confidence, commitment, conscience, or comportment—or Mayeroff's (1971) caring ingredients (knowing, patience, alternating rhythms, humility, hope, trust, honesty, or courage) are most important in this situation? How was the nurse and one nursed living caring, helping the other grow in her own time (Mayeroff, 1971)? Or was it humility, being open to know the other? What other expressions of caring, such as authentic presence, silence, or listening, were helpful?

Using the Ways of Knowing, How Can We Come to Understand the Call(s) for Nursing?

How does each of the ways of knowing—personal, empirical, ethical, sociopolitical, spiritual, emancipatory, unknowing, aesthetic—inform understanding of caring in this nursing situation (Carper, 1978; Kagen, Smith, Cowling, & Chinn, 2009; Munhall, 1993; White, 1995)?

Personal knowing: What do I need to know about myself and Sarah to care for her? Who am I as a caring person? How am I living caring as a student or professional nurse? Who is Sarah as a caring child? How is Sarah living caring? What personal knowledge do I bring to this situation? Do I know other children, relatives, and friends who have experienced this health concern? Have I ever cared for a child with this health concern before? What did I learn from that experience? How does that influence my caring in this unique situation?

Empirical knowing: What do I need to know about Sarah's health concerns to care for her? What can I bring from other disciplines to help me understand Sarah's unique situation and to care for her? What treatments has Sarah received? What have been her reactions to treatments, medications, and living with this health concern? What complementary modalities could be helpful and which ones has Sarah participated in? What was her reaction? What is the impact of Sarah's development stage on her understanding of her situation?

Ethical knowing: How should I care for this child? How do the values of the theoretical perspective guide nursing care in the right way for this child? How do professional ethical codes for nurses guide caring for Sarah? Am I honest with her? Am I keeping her personal information confidential?

Sociopolitical knowing: What is the context of this child's life, home, school, family, and friends? What environmental factors may have influenced her well-being? How would Sarah's health insurance coverage impact her health care (private pay, HMO, PPO, Medicaid)? What local, state, and federal policies and laws are impacting her well-being? What social structures impact the practice of nursing in this situation?

Spiritual knowing: How should I support this child's religious and/or spiritual beliefs and practices? What do I need to know?

Emancipatory knowing: How can the nurse care for Sarah in an environment of patriarchy? How can the nurse respond to any injustices about

Sarah's care? What injustices or power struggles between the child and the staff are present? What advocacy is needed in this situation?

Unknowing: What matters most to Sarah at this time? How should the nurse come to understand Sarah? How can the nurse bracket what is known about Sarah from the chart, report, or staff conversations and come to know her as a person uniquely living caring?

Aesthetic knowing: How can the nurse support Sarah's hopes and dreams? How can the nurse transcend this moment to create possibilities? How have the arts influenced knowing? What metaphors or artistic expressions could represent the caring between Sarah and the nurse in this situation? How does the nurse weave threads from all ways of knowing into the fabric of understanding caring in this nursing situation?

What Are the Calls for Nursing?

The nurse heard the call to be with Sarah on their shared journey. What are some possible variations in Sarah's calls for nursing?

What Are the Responses to the Calls for Nursing Present in the Situation?

The nurse responded to Sarah with authentic presence and appreciation of all that Sarah was. They became partners and they became friends, sharing smiles and jokes.

What were the expressions of caring? How did the ways of knowing inform caring? Which way of knowing was most informative? What are some possible variations in creating a response?

What Was the Outcome of the Response(s) in Relation to the Call(s)?

The nurse used the theoretical perspective of caring (FAU, CON, 2012) to focus on nurturing the wholeness and well-being of persons in caring relationships. In what way did the outcomes reflect this theoretical lens?

For the person nursed, Sarah: Sarah and her nurse were partners until her death. The nurse nurtured Sarah's wholeness by encouraging her artistic talents, her spirituality, and her way of being with people. Even though she was so young, she lived a life filled with meaning.

For the nurse: The nurse learned how to care from Sarah. She taught her how to live caring through patience, gratitude, presence, and unconditional love.

For the nursing profession: What can others learn about being a nurse and caring for a child with a terminal illness from this nursing situation? What can be learned about living with compassion and finding meaning in sad and sorrowful situations? What is the value of caring for and appreciating nurse colleagues?

For others: What is the value of being cared for? How can physicians, social workers, and other health care professionals learn from the generative nature of compassion?

How Did the Study of This Nursing Situation Enhance Your Knowledge of Nursing?

What did I learn about myself as I studied this situation? What did I learn about caring science? What new possibilities can be created from this nursing situation?

LEARNING ACTIVITIES

Journal: Reflect on and describe what happened between the nurse and one nursed.

BOX 12.1   Reflective Journal

What are your thoughts on caring expressed by the nurse in this situation?

Aesthetic re-presentation: How can this nursing situation be aesthetically re-presented?

BOX 12.2   Aesthetic Re-presentation

How would you aesthetically re-present this nursing situation?

REFERENCES

Carper, B. (1978). Fundamental patterns of knowing. *Advances in Nursing Science, 1*(1), 13–24.

Florida Atlantic University, Christine E. Lynn College of Nursing. (2012). *Philosophy*. Retrieved from http://nursing.fau.edu/index.php?main=1&nav=635

Kagen, P. N., Smith, M. C., Cowling, R., & Chinn, P. (2009). A nursing manifesto: An emancipatory call for nursing knowledge development, conscience, and practice. *Nursing Philosophy, 11*, 67–84.

Mayeroff, M. (1971). *On caring*. New York, NY: Harper Collins.

Munhall, P. (1993). Unknowing: Toward another pattern of knowing. *Nursing Outlook, 41*, 125–128.

Roach, S. (2002). *The human act of caring: A blueprint for the health professions* (2nd rev ed.). Ottawa, Canada: Canadian Hospital Association Press.

White, J. (1995). Patterns of knowing: Review, critique, and update. *Advances in Nursing Science, 17*(4), 73–86.

LEARNING RESOURCES

A Guide to End of Life Care. (2012). *Together for short lives*. Retrieved from http://www.togetherforshortlives.org.uk/assets/0000/1855/TfSL_A_Guide_to_End_of_Life_Care_5_FINAL_VERSION.pdf

American Nurses Association. (2010). *Registered nurses roles and responsibilities in providing expert care and counseling at the end of life: A position statement*. Silver Springs, MD: Author.

Boykin, A., & Schoenhofer, S. (1997). Reframing outcomes: Enhancing personhood. *Advanced Nursing Practice Quarterly, 3*(1), 60.

Smith, M. C. (2013). Caring and the discipline of nursing. In M. Smith, M. Turkel, & Z. Wolf (Eds.), *Caring in nursing classics: An essential resource* (pp. 1–8). New York, NY: Springer Publishing Co.

Weidner, N. J., Cameron, M., Lee, R., McBride, J., Mathias, E. J., & Byczkowski, T. L. (2011). End of life care for the dying child: What matters most to parents. *Journal of Palliative Care, 27*(4), 279–286.

CHAPTER 13

Caring Between a Nurse and a Group of Men Hospitalized With Chronic Mental Illness

This chapter presents a nursing situation focused on the caring between a nurse and a group of men hospitalized with chronic mental illness. The nurse used Watson's Theory of Human Caring (2010) as the broad theoretical lens that gives shape to his approach to nursing practice. This nursing situation highlights the transpersonal caring relationship between the nurse and the ones being cared for that creates harmony, wholeness, and unity of being in caring moments.

Directions: As you prepare to intentionally enter the world of the other, reflect on the following question: What are the expressions of caring between nurse and the one nursed?

NURSING SITUATION

Written by Michael Shaw, BSN, RN

4TH OF JULY PICNIC

Around the 4th of July, our large hospital provides a dazzling fireworks display for the local community. Everyone is invited and it is a fun-filled event geared toward employees, their families, and our patients. I wanted to do something special for the remaining eight patients that made up the psychiatric ward where I worked. This particular ward was being phased out and these eight men were considered "placement issues" because of the severity of their mental illness. The problem was, I work the A shift and the fireworks show was obviously scheduled in the evening. I began planning a party for the aforementioned men but, because of prior holiday commitments by the staff, found little support for my "party." Undaunted, I proceeded with my plans, eventually soliciting a few dollars.

At 7:00 p.m. the night of the celebration, I showed up with 10 large pizzas, five ice-cold watermelons, a cooler filled with soft drinks, lawn chairs, eight of the coolest-looking straw hats purchased at the local dollar store, and a boom-box with a Michael Jackson CD. We promptly set up folding tables in an open space outside the porch area of our ward that afforded an unobstructed view of the upcoming fireworks.

Let me just say we partied! The eight patients, three staff members, and I had a night to remember! The smiles on everyone's faces as we ate slice after slice of pizza and watermelon and danced to Michael Jackson hits remains a priceless memory. As I surveyed the scene, I was overcome by the feeling that this was more like a family reunion—we weren't just patients and staff members, but friends truly enjoying this special evening together.

Later, as darkness descended upon the grounds, a contented hush fell over our gathering in anticipation of the fireworks slated to begin. The show began, and besides the booming of the fireworks the only sound heard were the *ooohhs* and *aaaahhs* in appreciation of the fireworks that illuminated the evening sky.

Days later our ward would be closed and the patients dispersed, never to be seen or heard from again. As time passed, the glow of that wonderful evening would diminish and I would be transferred to another ward. Then one day as I was searching for an item in a storage closet, I happened across a funky little straw hat and the memories of that dancing while waiting for the fireworks to begin. Nursing is creating positive memories for your patients!

STUDY PROCESS

The Barry, Gordon & King Teaching/Learning Nursing Framework process is a broad guide to analyze the nursing situation, focusing on the caring concepts that bring nursing to life and the multiple ways of knowing needed to care for these men. Caring from Watson's Theory of Human Caring (2010) provides the inspiration for a new and different understanding of individuals.

What Was the Caring Between the Nurse and the One Nursed?

The nurse states we were present not as just staff members and patients, but as friends gathered for a party; we were there to serve, but not to order or direct our patients as we often do during the course of a normal work day. Also, we were not in uniform, which further broke down the divide between staff and patients. Actually, we were dressed in Hawaiian shirts and straw hats. We laughed and joked with our patients, even dancing with them or for them. The antiseptic atmosphere of their daily routine was replaced with one of relaxation and fun! Even the food we brought added to the festivities. Our patients rarely get to choose what they eat, especially different kinds of real pizza or sodas. "Can I have another one of those real Cokes?" asked one of our contented patients. Little things we take for granted were offered that evening to our party-goers. You should have seen the delight on their faces when we cut open several chilled watermelons. We had a blast with a seed spitting contest! We allowed ourselves to be free with our friends, unencumbered without the responsibility of observing, charting, monitoring, and so on.

What other expressions of caring did you identify as you read the nursing situation? What other caring concepts are present in the situation?

Using the Ways of Knowing, How Can We Come to Understand the Call(s) for Nursing?

How does each of the ways of knowing—personal, empirical, ethical, sociopolitical, spiritual, emancipatory, unknowing, aesthetic—inform understanding of caring in this nursing situation (Carper, 1978; Kagen, Smith, Cowling, & Chinn, 2009; Munhall, 1993; White, 1995)?

Personal knowing: How did the nurse's understanding of self as caring person support his understanding of others' expressions of caring? The nurse stated why he became a nurse:

> Remember why most of us got into nursing? It might sound cliché, but yeah, "I want to make a difference! Help people!" That's what we experienced that wonderful evening! Oh, the drudgery that sometimes make up our days as nurses—the meetings, the audits, in-services—but then, at any patient encounter, one can choose to make a difference! A smile, or kind word, just listening quietly to a concerned patient goes a tremendous way—and it is so simple to do! Never lose sight of what we are called to do! Remember receiving your first nursing degree, how excited we were, you were ready to conquer the world…we acted like new nurses that evening!

What other experiences or encounters of caring did the nurse bring to this nursing situation that helped him make such a difference in the lives of the men, his colleagues, and himself?

Empirical knowing: What does the nurse need to know about chronic mental illness? What research has been conducted on mental health and related topics of stigmatization and marginalization that contribute to understanding? How can the caring concepts of courage and compassion guide the nurse? How do Watson's caritas processes inspire transpersonal relationships? What does the nurse need to know about community resources to support transitions to community care?

Ethical knowing: How do codes for nurses provide a foundation for ethical practice? Which ethical principles grounded the nurse in acknowledging the dignity of this group of men and relating to them with respect? How should individuals with chronic mental illness be supported and cared for? How does the American Nurses Association Social Policy Statement (2010) enhance understanding of nursing roles, responsibility, and accountability in caring for vulnerable populations?

Sociopolitical knowing: What are the social determinants of health? How do they impact understanding of caring for vulnerable and marginalized groups? What are the local, state, and federal policies and laws that impact persons with mental illness?

Spiritual knowing: What faith-based resources are available in the community for persons with mental illness? Are there sources of spirituality that nurture the being of these men?

Emancipatory knowing: What is the role of nursing in advocating for the rights of persons with mental illness? What is the current status of health care parity for individuals with mental illness?

Unknowing: How can the nurse build trusting relationships with individuals with mental illness? How can the nurse uncover what matters most for each of these men?

Aesthetically knowing: How can the beauty of this nursing situation be re-presented in an art form? What other sources of knowledge would be helpful for you in caring for persons with mental illness?

What Are the Calls for Nursing?

The nurse heard a silent but distinct call from the men to be part of the mainstream community at the hospital. He states, "We were equals that night." What calls for nursing do you hear from this group of men?

What Are the Responses to the Calls for Nursing Present in the Situation?

The nurse created a party focused on giving these special men a chance to really enjoy themselves, just as if they were outside the facility's walls or at home. They could be loud, silly, eat as much as they wanted, and dance, whatever they wanted to do as long as they didn't harm themselves or others. It was their night! Also, the staff was not in uniform, but dressed in Hawaiian shirts and straw hats, which further broke down the divide between staff and patients. They laughed and joked with the patients, even dancing with them or for them. The antiseptic atmosphere of their daily routine was replaced with one of relaxation and fun! Even the food added to the festivities, as the patients rarely get to choose what they eat, especially different kinds of real pizza or sodas. "Can I have another one of those real Cokes?" asked one of the contented patients. Little things taken for granted were offered that evening to the party-goers. You should have seen the delight on their faces when several chilled watermelons were cut open. They had a blast with a seed spitting contest! The staff allowed themselves to be free with their friends, unencumbered without the responsibility of observing, charting, monitoring, and so on.

What are some possible variations in creating a response? How would you have responded using Watson's caritas processes?

What Was the Outcome of the Response(s) in Relation to the Call(s)?

The nurse used Watson's Theory of Human Caring (2010) and was inspired by certain caritas processes: the practice of loving kindness and equanimity, developing and sustaining a helping–trusting caring relationship, and the creative use of self. These caritas processes came together as an exquisite example of a transpersonal relationship that inspired a fun-filled caring occasion. The nurse later reflected that there under the stars and between brilliant flashes of fireworks booming overhead, a caring–healing–loving consciousness was formed. When the fireworks and party were over, the nurse reports that he witnessed something "very special, a column of men with arms around shoulders, giggling, laughing, and, yes, even belching as they brought this magical evening to a close."

For the nurse: The nurse later states,"I'm still in awe, we freed ourselves to allow love and caring to come together—we were not machines but spirits made whole."

For the ones nursed: The nurse reflected: "These lonely men felt like being part of a caring family for the first time in a long time. The feelings of being institutionalized evaporated for those few brief hours. Someone cared, someone responded to a need. The unselfish, kind acts of the staff that showed up that night! What a tremendous change in attitudes that occurred among the participants that evening."

For the staff: Caring has the potential to improve the well-being of persons. The nurse affirms this in his statement, "It certainly did on that one summer evening for the patients and staff assembled there; as it turned out, patients, this nurse, and staff were beneficiaries of this event."

For the nursing profession: This nursing situation is retold and offers untold opportunities for understanding anew the impact of caring from the lens of human caring. The focus of this theory is brought alive in this story as the participants experience harmony, wholeness, and unity of being in caring moments. The caring expressed is meaningful and beneficial for the nurse, the ones nursed, for the staff, colleagues, and for all who are drawn into this circle of universal caring.

For others: What is the value of being cared for? How does the nurse's story of this unique 4th of July picnic inspire hope for compassion for all persons, especially those who are particularly vulnerable such as those individuals living with mental illness?

How Did the Study of This Nursing Situation Enhance Your Knowledge of Nursing?

What did I learn about myself as I studied this situation? What did I learn about caring science? What new possibilities can be created from this nursing situation?

LEARNING ACTIVITIES

Journal: The outcomes of nursing situations cannot be predicted but can be imagined through thoughtful, intentional care. Reflect on and describe what happened between the nurse and the ones nursed.

BOX 13.1   Reflective Journal

What are your thoughts on caring expressed by the nurse in this situation?

Aesthetic re-presentation: How would you represent this nursing situation in an art form?

BOX 13.2   Aesthetic Re-presentation

How would you aesthetically re-present this nursing situation?

REFERENCES

American Nurses Association (ANA). (2010). *Social policy statement*. Silver Springs, MD: Author.

Carper, B. (1978). Fundamental patterns of knowing. *Advances in Nursing Science*, *1*(1), 13–24.

Florida Atlantic University, Christine E. Lynn College of Nursing. (2012). *Philosophy*. Retrieved from http://nursing.fau.edu/index.php?main=1&nav=635

Kagen, P. N., Smith, M. C., Cowling, R., & Chinn, P. (2009). A nursing manifesto: An emancipatory call for nursing knowledge development, conscience, and practice. *Nursing Philosophy*, *11*, 67–84.

Munhall, P. (1993). Unknowing: Toward another pattern of knowing. *Nursing Outlook*, *41*, 125–128.

Watson, J., & Woodward, T. K. (2010). Jean Watson's theory of human caring. In M. E. Parker & M. C. Smith (Eds.), *Nursing theories and nursing practice* (3rd ed., pp. 351–369). Philadelphia, PA: F.A. Davis.

White, J. (1995). Patterns of knowing: Review, critique, and update. *Advances in Nursing Science*, *17*(4), 73–86.

LEARNING RESOURCES

DeSilva, M., Samele, C., Sacena, S., Patel, V., & Darzi, A. (2014). Policy actions to achieve integrated community-based mental health services. *Health Affairs*, *33*(9), 1595–1602.

National Institute of Mental Health. (2015). Transforming the understanding and treatment of mental illnesses. Retrieved from http://www.nimh.nih.gov/index.shtml

Ryan, L. (2005). The journey to integrate Watson's caring theory with clinical practice. *International Journal for Human Caring*, *9*(3), 26–30.

Townsend, M. C. (2011). *Psychiatric mental health nursing: Concepts of care in evidenced based practice*. Philadelphia, PA: F.A. Davis.

Yang, L. H., Chen, F., Sia, K. J., Lam, J., Lam, K., Ngo, H., . . . Good, B. (2014). "What matters most?" A cultural mechanism moderating structural vulnerability & moral experience of mental health stigma. *Social Science & Medicine*, *103*, 84–93.

CHAPTER 14

Caring Between a Nurse and an Adult Transitioning From Acute Care to Home Care

This chapter presents a nursing situation focused on caring of a young adult male admitted with chest pain and his nurse. Using the philosophical perspective of caring (Florida Atlantic University, Christine E. Lynn College of Nursing [FAU, CON], 2012), which focuses on nurturing the wholeness and well-being of persons in caring relationships, the nursing situation highlights the nurse's growing understanding of caring.

Directions: As you prepare to intentionally enter the world of the other, reflect on the following question: What are the expressions of caring between nurse and the one nursed?

NURSING SITUATION

WRITTEN BY SHELINA DAVIS, ARNP, GNP-BC

BOB AND HIS DOGS

Recently, I met a young male who presented to the emergency department with chest pain. I will just call him Bob. He underwent a cardiac catheterization and was found to have severe multivessel coronary artery disease and was referred to the cardiothoracic surgical team. I introduced myself to the small-framed gentleman and began to talk to him and ask him my usual questions. He rested on the recovery stretcher, very relaxed and very attentive to everything I explained. He asked questions along the way and seemed very accepting of (a) his newly diagnosed severe artery disease, (b) learning that he was a poor candidate for nonsurgical revascularization, and (c) being told that surgeons were prepared to take him for bypass grafting the next morning! I remember Bob coming to his decision rather quickly without any vacillation or discernible trepidation. The more I explained, the more eager he was to learn more.

After almost 2 hours of speaking with Bob and getting to know him, I learned he was a bit of a loner. He had never been married. His family lived in another state and he had not seen them in years. However, he had neighbors that were willing to help him at any time. I wrapped up the consult and began preparing him for the day's events. I remember thinking to myself how unusual this was for me because I normally would have needed more time for patients and family members to think and digest everything. Not Bob! By his verbal and nonverbal cues, I could tell he was ready for more. He was open to every aspect of his hospital stay that I discussed—from preoperative testing to discharge home—and accepting of things to come. I ended my extended visit with Bob and I asked him if there was anything we had not covered that was important to him or any questions that I had not answered or needed clearing up. He smiled widely and replied, "Nope. I think I am ready." He went off to surgery the next day.

Bob did very well postoperatively. I saw him every day throughout his recovery and continued to build a solid patient–provider relationship with him. He was discharged on postoperative day six with a follow-up scheduled in the office to see me. He presented for his first postoperative visit and had developed drainage, swelling, and pain at the distal end of his sternal incision. I opened the incision by sterile technique and realized the area of drainage was very large. I admitted him back into the hospital for incision and drainage of the entire area. Through it all, again, he was a trooper. A wound vacuum system was placed on the wound in the operating room and I saw him the next morning. I felt very good about his short stay and was even more excited that all had gone so well. Besides, I had more teaching to share about things to come.

Just as I had done before, I explained to him everything to come. I explained that he would go home with the wound vacuum system and that nurses would come in every other day to change the foam packing. This time he was very quiet. I continued on without missing a beat. Later that evening, I briefly thought about him but I wasn't sure why. By the end of the week, postoperative day three, he was scheduled for discharge. As the nurse was preparing Bob for discharge, he began to have chest pains. Diagnostic testing was unrevealing and he was monitored over the weekend. I made rounds on Monday morning and Bob seemed to be doing very well. I reviewed everything that happened over the weekend and I began to recall my last encounter with Bob. Therefore, I decided to hang around for a couple of hours.

Later his nurse began to go over discharge information with him and he began to complain of chest pain and dizziness. I entered the room and he looked terrified. He was pale, very fearful, and avoiding eye contact. He looked nothing like the Bob I had come to know. I asked the nurse to give us some time and I sat down beside him and we began to talk. Eventually he revealed how he could not go home. He expressed how he felt no fear facing his own mortality after being diagnosed with severe coronary disease and undergoing open-heart surgery. He continued to tell me that everything had gone just as he had learned through my teaching. He felt no fear until I told him that nurses would come into his home to do dressing changes. As it turns out, Bob had two dogs that were deemed very aggressive. He knew he could not have anyone in his home, but he didn't know how to tell me. He didn't know that he had options. He was afraid that his dogs would suffer as a result of his care needs and feared that they may be taken away.

I realized then that I had missed something very special with Bob. His dogs were his close family. His dogs loved, comforted, and protected him. With them, he had no fears and felt he would be fine at home. Due to his special needs, I made arrangements for Bob to come into my office Monday, Wednesday, and Friday for dressing changes. He was very thankful, and so was I. He taught me a valuable lesson.

Within half an hour, Bob was chasing the nurse down the hall for discharge information, asking questions, and being very attentive to his instructions for skin care and managing the wound vacuum system. He went home that afternoon and continued to eagerly learn as he recovered from his surgical experience. Nursing is learning and connecting to what matters most to the patient and trying to make health care fit his or her needs; the care of the patient affects his or her experience in health, illness, and recovery.

STUDY PROCESSES

The Barry, Gordon & King Teaching/Learning Nursing Framework process is a broad guide to study and analyze nursing situations, focusing on the caring between the nurse and one nursed. In caring for Bob, the nurse followed her routine of educating Bob prior to surgery and following up with discharge teaching. The following analysis guides and inspires understanding of nursing from the philosophical perspective of caring (FAU, CON, 2012), focusing on nurturing the wholeness and well-being of persons in caring relationships.

What Was the Caring Between the Nurse and the One Nursed?

The nurse cared for Bob through her competent teaching about his surgery and discharge care. She was committed to understanding why Bob became symptomatic each time he was getting close to being discharged. As the nurse realized that Bob was telling her something, she became more fully present and he shared his concern about strangers coming into his home and his fear of losing his family—his dogs. The nurse genuinely listened to Bob and trust had been established. What mattered most in the moment to Bob? What other caring ingredients are present in the situation? How did the nurse instill trust with the one nursed? How did the nurse's competence influence the situation?

Using the Ways of Knowing, How Can We Understand the Call(s) for Nursing?

How does each of the ways of knowing—personal, empirical, ethical, sociopolitical, spiritual, emancipatory, unknowing, and aesthetic—inform understanding of caring in this nursing situation (Carper, 1978; Kagen, Smith, Cowling, & Chinn, 2009; Munhall, 1993; White, 1995)?

Personal knowing: What is conveyed by the nurse and Bob as a caring person? What can be learned from Bob regarding the definition of family? What past experiences with aggressive dogs might influence the nurse's caring? What do you need to know about yourself to care for Bob?

Empirical knowing: What knowledge is needed to provide nursing care for a person undergoing a coronary bypass surgery? What knowledge is needed to care for a person with a wound vacuum system? What is the research related to preventive measures for coronary heart disease? What is the influence of a person's mental health on physical health? What does Bob need to know as he transitions from the acute care setting to his home? What evidence informs transitional care? What knowledge of family theory is needed to care for Bob? What are the laws for animals that are designated aggressive?

Ethical knowing: What ethical issues are present in this nursing situation? How do ethical codes guide nursing practice? Who should pay for the additional hospital stays?

Sociopolitical knowing: What is the sociological impact of coronary artery disease? What preventative health measures are covered by insurance companies? What are the cost comparisons between in-home and in-office postoperative wound care? How does Bob's cultural belief impact his health? What measures could be taken to assist Bob with his dogs labeled as aggressive?

Spiritual knowing: How can the nurse support Bob's spiritual beliefs and practices?

Emancipatory knowing: What bureaucratic constraints are present in this nursing situation? What advocacy actions are needed?

Unknowing: What mattered most in the moment to Bob? What must it be like for Bob to live in fear that his dogs will be taken away from him?

What did the nurse unknowingly communicate to Bob through her actions and communication?

Aesthetic knowing: How did the nurse support Bob's hopes and dreams? How would you aesthetically represent this nursing situation?

What Are the Calls for Nursing?

The nurse heard the call to provide patient teaching and education for Bob regarding his coronary artery disease, bypass surgery, and postoperative care. She also heard his call to understand his fear of losing his family (dogs). What other calls would you identify in this nursing situation?

What Are the Responses to the Calls for Nursing Present in the Situation?

The nurse initially responded to the call for education and patient teaching, but once she listened she addressed his issue with home care. What other responses might you create? What expressions of caring are present? How did the ways of knowing inform the nurse's response? Which way of knowing was most informative in the responses?

What Was the Outcome of the Response(s) in Relation to the Call(s)?

The nurse used the philosophical perspective of caring (FAU, CON, 2012), which focuses on nurturing the wholeness and well-being of persons in caring relationships. In what way did the outcomes reflect this theoretical lens?

For the person nursed, Bob: What mattered most to Bob was his family— his dogs. He was fearful of transitioning to home care because of his dogs' past behavior with strangers. As plans for him to receive care at the nurse's office evolved, his fears were allayed and he was now eager to go home.

For the nurse: The nurse learned to be more fully present through active listening and realized the need to make health care fit the person's unique circumstance.

For the nursing profession: This nursing situation exemplifies the uniqueness of calls and responses and the need for nurses to listen to each individual and what matters most to the person at that moment in time.

For others: What is the value of being cared for? What is the value of understanding the meaning of family? How does coming to know an individual facilitate economical transitional care?

How Did the Study of This Nursing Situation Enhance Your Knowledge of Nursing?

What did I learn about myself as I studied this situation? What did I learn about caring science? What new possibilities can be created from this nursing situation?

LEARNING ACTIVITIES

Journal: Reflect on the importance of knowing others through active listening and authentic presence. Write a nursing situation from your practice exemplifying the value of understanding what matters most to the person.

BOX 14.1   Reflective Journal

What are your thoughts on caring expressed by the nurse in this situation?

Aesthetic re-presentation: How can this nursing situation be aesthetically re-presented?

BOX 14.2   Aesthetic Re-presentation

How would you aesthetically re-present this nursing situation?

REFERENCES

Carper, B. (1978). Fundamental patterns of knowing. *Advances in Nursing Science, 1*(1), 13–24.

Florida Atlantic University, Christine E. Lynn College of Nursing. (2012). *Philosophy.* Retrieved from http://nursing.fau.edu/index.php?main=1&nav=635

Kagen, P. N., Smith, M. C., Cowling, R., & Chinn, P. (2009). A nursing manifesto: An emancipatory call for nursing knowledge development, conscience, and practice. *Nursing Philosophy, 11,* 67–84.

Munhall, P. (1993). Unknowing: Toward another pattern of knowing. *Nursing Outlook, 41*, 125–128.

White, J. (1995). Patterns of knowing: Review, critique, and update. *Advances in Nursing Science, 17*(4), 73–86.

LEARNING RESOURCES

Browning, S., & Waite, R. (2010). The gift of listening: JUST listening strategies. *Nursing Forum, 45*(3), 150–158.

Centers for Medicare and Medicaid Services. (2015). Community-based transitional care programs. Retrieved from http://innovation.cms.gov/initiatives/CCTP/

Initiative on the Future of Nursing. (2011). Transitional care model. Retrieved from http://thefutureofnursing.org/resource/detail/transitional-care-model

McMahon, M., & Christopher, K. (2011). Toward a mid-range theory of nursing presence. *Nursing Forum, 46*(2), 71–82.

Meleis, A. I. (2010). *Transitions theory: Middle-range and situation-specific theories in nursing research and practice.* New York, NY: Springer Publishing.

Turkell, M. (2001). Struggling to find a balance: The paradox between caring and economics. *Nursing Administration Quarterly, 26*(1), 67–82.

CHAPTER 15

Caring Between a Nurse Practitioner and an Adult Living With End-Stage Kidney Disease Transitioning to Home Care

This chapter presents a nursing situation focused on the caring between an adult living with end-stage kidney disease (ESKD) and a nurse practitioner. Using the perspective of Story Theory (Smith & Liehr, 2010), the nursing situation highlights the nature of caring for an adult living with ESKD. The theory guides the nurse practitioner in discovering what matters most to the person, connecting with the individual, and creating moments of ease as the one nursed moves toward resolving his health challenge.

Directions: As you prepare to intentionally enter the world of the other, reflect on the following question: What are the expressions of caring between nurse practitioner and the one nursed?

NURSING SITUATION

Written by Debra Hain, PhD, ARNP, ANP-BC, GNP-BC, FAANP

INTENTIONAL DIALOGUE TO DISCOVER WHAT MATTERS MOST

James is a 40-year-old African American male who has end-stage kidney disease (ESKD) and is receiving hemodialysis at a free-standing dialysis center for 4 hours three times a week. Three months ago he started dialysis for a second time. Twelve years ago he had undergone hemodialysis for 2 years before he received a kidney transplant. A recent rejection of the kidney transplant led to initiating hemodialysis once again. I have cared for people undergoing dialysis for over 25 years and although they have similar medical diagnoses, each person comes with unique gifts to be shared in the person–nurse relationship.

I visit James at the dialysis center three times a month. During most visits James appears to be hypervigilant as he watches every move the dialysis staff (nurses and dialysis technicians) make. On one occasion, as I intentionally engaged in dialogue with James about the challenges he faces, he disclosed his lack of trust for staff at the center. In turn, the dialysis staff expressed that James "is a difficult patient." Negative emotions have resulted in a task-oriented approach to "get the treatment done in a timely and safe manner" so James can go home. The nurses and dialysis technicians have demonstrated technological competence; however, I wonder, based on his concerns, if the staff sees James as an extension of the machine or the machine as an extension of James. Is the care focused on the technology rather than on James as a person?

James told his story of when he was on dialysis 12 years ago, how his wife had died, and how, just when he was fortunate to find a new love and have another child, his body rejected his transplant and he had to restart dialysis. As his story unfolded I sensed his pain, anguish, and bewilderment of the here and now and what the future may bring. How does all of this fit in his future hopes and dreams of being a father to his son and becoming an author of a motivational book for people living with ESKD? Our dialogue moved beyond a therapeutic medical conversation to a caring dialogue where the nurse cares enough to truly listen to what is being said and what is not being said.

The nurse and the one nursed experience connectedness—a sense of oneness. James trusts the nurse enough to disclose his fears of the staff making another error, for this had happened in past hemodialysis treatments before his kidney transplant. Some dialysis centers reuse dialyzers that are specific to one person and undergo sterilization after each treatment until the filter is no longer effective in removing toxins and waste products. On one occasion, while preparing the machine for James's treatment, a technician made an error and used another person's dialyzer; the other person had hepatitis B and was HIV positive. Follow-up laboratory tests were congruent with James's awareness that it was unlikely he would be infected with these diseases; however, the psychological impact was almost more than he could bear.

Further dialogue revealed James's strong desire to be actively involved in care decisions. Realizing this, I knew the importance of ensuring that he was aware of contemporary treatment modalities that have emerged in the past few years. I identified that he had no knowledge about the newest form of home hemodialysis. This treatment modality promotes one's ability to play a key role as a member of the health care team because individuals manage their treatment at home with remote guidance from expert nurses. At first James was skeptical; to decrease his anxiety related to the new modality, I recommended that he meet other people involved in home hemodialysis. Even though he expressed concern about his current care environment, he was not ready to consider another modality. I assured him that I would be with him on his journey and when he was ready to contemplate this option I would be happy to assist him in determining the best treatment options for him.

Months later, he experienced an episode of hypotension and light-headedness during dialysis. He told the nurse he didn't feel good and she responded with the usual nursing intervention without individualizing his care. The intervention didn't resolve the problem as it recurred several times over the next 2 weeks. The nurse thought that James was anxious and needed medication to calm him. I spoke with James and he replied, "I don't think I am anxious, I just don't feel good." His comments made me consider possible reasons for his symptoms and further investigation revealed an electrolyte imbalance, which was easily addressed. His symptoms were resolved, but the distrust for the dialysis staff increased.

Once again James and I engaged in dialogue about home hemodialysis and this time James agreed to look into it. I met James at the center where people are trained and partner with the nursing staff to manage home hemodialysis. After meeting people receiving home hemodialysis and talking with the nurses caring for these people, he decided to try this modality. Six months later, I met with James again and he enthusiastically exclaimed, "I am so happy; this was the best option for me!" He was able to spend time with his son and achieve his dream of authoring a book. He wrote a book about his experiences of living with ESKD and included messages of hope for others with ESKD. Currently, James is undergoing an evaluation for another kidney transplant and living life to the fullest.

STUDY PROCESSES

The Barry, Gordon & King Teaching/Learning Nursing Framework process is a broad guide to study and analyze nursing situations, focusing on the caring between the nurse and one nursed. In caring for James the nurse practitioner reaches out from inside the core of the nursing situation to the periphery to explore particular caring concepts that bring the situation to life; to find relevant characteristics of the person, nurse, and environment unique to the situation; and to examine the advanced knowledge needed to care for a person with ESKD. The following analysis will guide and inspire understanding of nursing from the theoretical perspective of story (Smith & Liehr, 2010), focusing on creating ease and movement toward resolving a health challenge.

What Was the Caring Between the Nurse and the One Nursed?

The nurse practitioner states, "Our dialogue moved beyond a therapeutic medical conversation to a caring dialogue where the nurse practitioner cares enough to truly listen to what is being said and what is not being said." The nurse practitioner and person nursed experience connectedness, a sense of oneness. James trusts the nurse enough to disclose his fears of the staff making another error, for this had happened in past hemodialysis treatments before his kidney transplant.

What caring concepts opened the door for the nurse practitioner to discover what matters most to James? What caring components from Roach (1987/2002)—competence, compassion, confidence, commitment, conscience, or comportment—or Mayeroff's (1971) caring ingredients (knowing, patience, alternating rhythms, humility, hope, trust, honesty, or courage) are the most important in this situation? Were there other expressions of caring that were helpful in this nursing situation?

Using the Ways of Knowing, How Can We Come to Understand the Call(s) for Nursing?

How does each of the ways of knowing—personal, empirical, ethical, socio-political, spiritual, emancipatory, unknowing, aesthetic—inform understanding of caring in this nursing situation (Carper, 1978; Kagen, Smith, Cowling, & Chinn, 2009; Munhall, 1993; White, 1995)?

Personal knowing: What do I need to know about myself when caring for a person with ESKD and receiving kidney replacement therapy (KRT)? Who am I as a caring person? How am I living caring as a student or professional nurse? Who is this adult as a caring person? How is this adult living caring? What personal knowledge do I bring to this situation? Do I know other adults with ESKD—relatives or friends who have experienced hemodialysis or other forms of KRT? Have I ever cared for a person with kidney disease receiving KRT in the past or someone who experienced a rejection of his kidney transplant? What do I know about having more than one kidney transplant? Who is eligible and who is not? What did I learn from that experience?

How does that influence my caring in this unique situation? How could I be present for others considering the best KRT options for them?

Empirical knowing: What does the nurse need to know about ESKD and KRT? How can other disciplines help inform understanding of James? How can the nurse help James understand his options for kidney replacement? What is home hemodialysis? What health challenges related to ESKD can people have? What symptoms are related to the dialysis treatment and how are they treated? What does technological competency mean? How can technological competency be expressed as caring? Identify caring behaviors that demonstrate competence and comportment as attributes of caring. What KRT choices does an adult with ESKD have? How can the nurse move beyond viewing a person receiving KRT as an object of his or her care toward knowing the individual as whole and complete in the moment?

Ethical knowing: What are the nurse's ethical obligations in this nursing situation and what should be done? How should the nurse demonstrate to others that James is a caring person? How can meaningful relationships between the dialysis staff and James provide support, respect, and caring? What are the ethical issues to consider when discussing kidney transplant with a person? Who is eligible for transplant? Who is not eligible for a kidney transplant? How does the nurse discuss eligibility with individuals who live with the future hope of receiving a kidney transplant?

Sociopolitical knowing: What is the ESKD program that is funded by Centers of Medicare and Medicaid? Who is eligible for the benefit? Can people receiving KRT continue to work? How can the nurse collaborate with other members of the health care team to support James in achieving his hopes and dreams? Who are his family members? Kidney disease recently has been recognized as a public health problem; how does the nurse increase awareness of risks of kidney disease at local, national, and global levels? What social structures impact the practice of nursing in this situation? How can the nurse be culturally sensitive to attend to the unique needs of each person?

Spiritual knowing: How does the nurse discover James's religious and/or spiritual beliefs and practices? How should the nurse support James's religious and/or spiritual beliefs and practices? How is James comforted spiritually? With whom on the team can the nurse collaborate to meet James's spiritual needs?

Emancipatory knowing: How can the nurse care for an individual in an environment that is driven by technology? How can the nurse respond to any injustices the person may feel about care or life in general? What injustices or power struggles are evident between a person receiving in-center hemodialysis and the dialysis staff? What advocacy is needed and how can the nurse advocate for both the nurse and one nursed in this situation? How can the nurse promote shared decision making that recognizes the person has the right to be involved in decisions about KRT such as dialysis modality choice, kidney transplant, or palliative care? How does the nurse find information about organ donation and allocation? Who can be a donor? How are kidney donors classified? How will kidney transplant candidates be classified? What happens to a person whose organ type is difficult to match? What happens to older adults and children?

Unknowing: How should the nurse come to understand the person with ESKD? How can the nurse bracket what is known about the person with ESKD from the medical record or the dialysis machine, while coming to know the individual uniquely living caring in this situation? What does the nurse learn from the person with ESKD from unknowing effort? How does the nurse discover what matters most at the present moment? What are James's future hopes and dreams?

Aesthetic knowing: How can the nurse support a person's hopes and dreams? How is caring creatively expressed in this situation? How can art and music influence emotional health? How can the nurse be present with James as he embraces his dream of writing a book? How is caring aesthetically expressed in this nursing situation? What complementary modalities can be used to ease a person's symptoms in a dialysis center?

What Are the Calls for Nursing?

The nurse practitioner heard James's call to be understood and to be cared for competently. What variations in the call(s) for nursing do you hear?

What Are the Responses to the Calls for Nursing Present in the Situation?

The nurse practitioner spent time with James and listened to his fears about contamination or other possible errors without judgment. She asked him if he would be interested in home dialysis and he jumped at the chance to be home, feel safe, and spend more time with his son. The nurse practitioner facilitated this process for him and in doing so created ease in his movement toward managing his ongoing kidney care. What are some variations in responses to the call(s) for nursing?

What Was the Outcome of the Response(s) in Relation to the Call(s)?

The nurse used the theoretical perspective of story (Smith & Liehr, 2010) that focuses on creating ease as the person moves toward resolving a health challenge. In what way did the outcomes reflect this theoretical lens?

For the person nursed, James: He wanted to be well, lead a full life, and write a book about his situation. And he did. He was so happy that he had begun hemodialysis. He was spending time with his son and felt well enough to write the book he dreamed about. As the story unfolds, James is considering another transplant.

For the advanced practice nurse: The nurse practitioner experienced the positive impact caring for James had on him and his family and was gratified by the outcomes. She learned how to establish trust in a person who had lost trust in the health care team and learned the usefulness of Story Theory to guide advanced practice focused on attending to what matters most for the one nursed.

For the nursing profession: Retelling this nursing situation for teaching/ learning purposes provides evidence of the power of caring science to reframe outcomes that are positive, and to support the other's hopes and dreams of flourishing while living with a chronic health concern.

For others: What is the value of being cared for? What is the value of witnessing James being cared for so thoughtfully and patiently for the team of nurses, technicians, and doctors? What can be learned about committing to be present, build trust, and watch the person flourish? What can be learned from the nurse practitioner's leadership in managing care?

How Did the Study of This Nursing Situation Enhance Your Knowledge of Nursing?

What did I learn about myself as I studied this situation? What did I learn about caring science? What new possibilities can be created from this nursing situation?

LEARNING ACTIVITIES

Journal: Reflect on and describe what happened between the nurse and one nursed.

BOX 15.1   Reflective Journal

What are your thoughts on caring expressed by the nurse in this situation?

Aesthetic re-presentation: How can the beauty of this nursing situation be re-presented in an aesthetic way?

BOX 15.2   Aesthetic Re-presentation

How would you aesthetically re-present this nursing situation?

REFERENCES

Carper, B. (1978). Fundamental patterns of knowing. *Advances in Nursing Science, 1*(1), 13–24.

Florida Atlantic University, Christine E. Lynn College of Nursing. (2012). *Philosophy*. Retrieved from http://nursing.fau.edu/index.php?main=1&nav=635

Kagen, P. N., Smith, M. C., Cowling, R., & Chinn, P. (2009). A nursing manifesto: An emancipatory call for nursing knowledge development, conscience, and practice. *Nursing Philosophy, 11,* 67–84.

Mayeroff, M. (1971). *On caring*. New York, NY: Harper Collins.

Munhall, P. (1993). Unknowing: Toward another pattern of knowing. *Nursing Outlook, 41,* 125–128.

Roach, M. S. (1987/2002). *Caring, the human mode of being: A blueprint for the health professions (2nd rev. ed.)*. Ottawa, Canada: The Canadian Hospital Association Press.

Smith, M. J., & Liehr, P. (2010). Story theory. In M. Parker & M. Smith (Eds.), *Nursing theories & nursing practice* (3rd ed., pp. 439–450). Philadelphia, PA: F.A. Davis.

White, J. (1995). Patterns of knowing: Review, critique, and update. *Advances in Nursing Science, 17*(4), 73–86.

LEARNING RESOURCES

American Nephrology Nurses Association. (2014). Retrieved from www.annanurse.org

Doss-McQuitty, S. (2012). Alternative dialysis therapies--why all the interest? *Nephrology Nursing Journal: Journal of the American Nephrology Nurses' Association, 40*(1), 17–20.

Hain, D. J., & Sandy, D. (2012). Partners in care: Patient empowerment through shared decision making. *Nephrology Nursing Journal: Journal of the American Nephrology Nurses' Association, 40*(2), 153–157.

Hain, D. J., Wands, L., & Liehr, P. (2011). Approaches to resolve health challenges in a population of older adults undergoing hemodialysis. *Research in Gerontological Nursing, 4*(1), 53–62.

International Transplant Nurses Society. (2013). About International Transplant Nurses Society. Retrieved from http://www.itns.org/About/About/aboutitns.html

National Kidney Foundation. (2013). Retrieved from www.kidney.org

Russell, C. L. (2013). Optimal care for kidney transplant recipients. *OR Nurse 2014, 7*(1), 36–40.

Sheu, J., Ephraim, P. L., Powe, N. R., Rabb, H., Senga, M., Evans, K. E., & Boulware, L. E. (2012). African American and non-African American patients' and families' decision making about renal replacement therapies. *Qualitative Health Research, 22*(7), 997–1006.

United Network for Organ Sharing (UNOS; 2015). Vision, mission & values. Retrieved from http://www.unos.org/about/index.php?topic=vision_mission_values

Weng, L. C., Dai, Y. T., Huang, H. L., & Chiang, Y. J. (2010). Self-efficacy, self-care behaviours and quality of life of kidney transplant recipients. *Journal of Advanced Nursing, 66*(4), 828–838.

CHAPTER 16

Caring Between a Nurse and an Older Adult Male in a Long-Term Care Setting

This chapter presents a nursing situation focused on the caring between a nurse and an older adult male in a long-term care setting. Using the philosophical perspective of caring (FAU, CON, 2012), which focuses on nurturing the wholeness and well-being of persons in caring relationships, the nursing situation highlights the nurse's growing understanding of caring.

Directions: As you prepare to intentionally enter the world of the other, reflect on the following question: What are the expressions of caring between nurse and the one nursed?

NURSING SITUATION

Written by Alina Miracle, DNP, ARNP, FNP-C

A DATE FOR DANCING

My nursing situation occurred when I worked at a long-term care facility. One morning during report I heard loud voices from one of the rooms. A nurse explained that Mr. Nuñez was combative during morning care and warned me that he usually refused care and his medications. That morning he told me to get out of his room and would not take his pills. While I was there I commented on the music his roommate was playing and Mr. Nuñez told me he liked the Glenn Miller Orchestra because he and his wife used to dance to his music.

That morning, the activity staff was playing music in the dining room and I noticed Mr. Nuñez coming in and out of his room asking anyone that walked by to dance; his approach was brusque and loud and no one would dance with him. He came to me and told me he liked the Glenn Miller Orchestra music better, so I told him I would see if I could get some of their music for him. That afternoon when I gave him his medication he refused and I told him I would be back in a few minutes. When I returned I told him about the evening activities and encouraged him to go. At that time during our conversation he reached for the medicine cup in my hand and took his medicines.

The next day after he finished breakfast I told him I had the music he liked and played the CD for him. As soon as the music started playing he stood up and began dancing with an imaginary partner. It was then that I noticed him smiling—he rarely did that. Later that morning he took his medications without any problems. We had a short conversation and he asked me if I would dance with him; pointing to the clock I told him that we could dance at 2 p.m. During the morning he stopped by the nurses' station frequently and reminded me of my promise.

At 2 p.m. I played his favorite song and we danced to his special song. He kept saying throughout the song that he used to dance with his wife to this song and how much he loves dancing. That afternoon he took his medications without any problems but later I heard him yelling at the staff, so I went in the room and explained that he needed to be cleaned up and he accepted my help and complied without question.

From that day on, every day that I worked he would ask me if we were going to dance at 2 p.m. and I would try my best to make time for Mr. Nuñez and dance with him. The time we interacted made me feel closer to this resident and I looked forward to our 2 p.m. dance. Just seeing how happy this small gesture made him reinforced one of the reasons why I went into nursing and geriatrics—the ability to make a difference in someone's life. Afterward, he would tell everyone that he had danced and kept the CD in his room like it was his greatest treasure.

STUDY PROCESSES

The Barry, Gordon & King Teaching/Learning Nursing Framework process is a broad guide to study and analyze nursing situations, focusing on the caring between the nurse and one nursed. In caring for Mr. Nuñez, the nurse realized how she could make such a difference in a person's life by a simple act of caring. The following analysis guides and inspires understanding of nursing from the philosophical perspective of caring (FAU, CON, 2012), focusing on nurturing the wholeness and well-being of persons in caring relationships.

What Was the Caring Between the Nurse and the One Nursed?

The nurse stated that interacting with Mr. Nuñez made her feel closer to him and that she looked forward to their 2 p.m. dance, and that seeing how happy this small gesture of listening and being authentically present made a difference in his life created meaning for Mr. Nuñez and for herself. What other expressions of caring are present in this nursing situation?

Using the Ways of Knowing, How Can We Come to Understand the Call(s) for Nursing?

How does each of the ways of knowing—personal, empirical, ethical, sociopolitical, spiritual, emancipatory, unknowing, aesthetic—inform understanding of caring in this nursing situation (Carper, 1978; Kagen, Smith, Cowling, & Chinn, 2009; Munhall, 1993; White, 1995)?

Personal knowing: How did the nurse live caring by having the courage to dance? How did Mr. Nuñez live caring by speaking out and taking the chance to dance? How will this experience deepen my understanding of finding courage to step out of the box and create possibilities for caring?

Empirical knowing: What knowledge is needed to care for a person with beginning dementia? The complementary modalities of music and dance were helpful for Mr. Nuñez; what are other possibilities? What therapeutic communication techniques would be beneficial to enhancing the wholeness and well-being of Mr. Nuñez? What nursing best practices and knowledge from other disciplines could enhance understanding persons with dementia?

Ethical knowing: How did the theoretical lens guide the nurse's ethical practice? What is the meaning of the ethical principle of fidelity and how is keeping promises lived in this nursing situation? How do codes of ethics guide nursing practice?

Spiritual knowing: How could the nurse support Mr. Nuñez's spiritual beliefs and practices?

Sociopolitical knowing: How do Mr. Nuñez's cultural beliefs impact his health and well-being? Who are his family members and friends? Do they live nearby or at a distance? What relationship does Mr. Nuñez have with staff members?

Unknowing: How could the nurse remain open to understanding Mr. Nuñez's hopes and dreams?

Emancipatory knowing: What are the rules and regulations that govern extended care facilities? How would existing policies affect Mr. Nuñez's wholeness and well-being? How could interprofessional collaboration ensure Mr. Nuñez's music and dance interactions continue when the nurse is not present at the long-term care facility?

Aesthetic knowing: What is the beauty of nursing in this nursing situation? How could this nursing situation be re-presented aesthetically?

What Are the Calls for Nursing?

The nurse states that through Mr. Nuñez's shouting she heard a silent call to help him relive old memories of dancing with his wife to swing music. She understood that the symbolic meaning of music and dance mattered most to him at that time. What other calls may be present?

What Are the Responses to the Calls for Nursing Present in the Situation?

The nurse responded to the call for nursing with courage and commitment to find some old swing music and to make a date to dance with him every day at 2 p.m. What other nursing responses could be created?

What Was the Outcome of the Response(s) in Relation to the Call(s)?

The author used the philosophical perspective of caring (FAU, CON, 2012), which focuses on nurturing the wholeness and well-being of persons in caring relationships.

For the person nursed, Mr. Nuñez: What mattered most for Mr. Nuñez was honored and celebrated in his daily dance to Glenn Miller's music. He was transformed by this simple gesture of caring.

For the nurse: The nurse was also transformed by this date for dancing and decided to specialize in caring for older adults.

For the nursing profession: The discipline and professional practice of nursing are also transformed by the retelling and sharing of this nursing situation that illuminates the value of caring so simply.

For others: What is the value of being cared for? Caring witnessed by other health care workers at the long-term facility reawakens appreciation for the beauty in simple acts of caring.

How Did the Study of This Nursing Situation Enhance Your Knowledge of Nursing?

What did I learn about myself as I studied this situation? What did I learn about caring science? What new possibilities can be created from this nursing situation?

LEARNING ACTIVITIES

Journal: Reflect on this nursing situation and how authentic presence, courage, and music nurtured wholeness and well-being. What happened between the nurses and Mr. Nuñez?

BOX 16.1   Reflective Journal

What are your thoughts on caring expressed by the nurse in this situation?

Aesthetic re-presentation: How can this nursing situation be aesthetically re-presented?

BOX 16.2   Aesthetic Re-presentation

How would you aesthetically re-present this nursing situation?

REFERENCES

Carper, B. (1978). Fundamental patterns of knowing. *Advances in Nursing Science, 1*(1), 13–24.

Florida Atlantic University, Christine E. Lynn College of Nursing. (2012). *Philosophy.* Retrieved from http://nursing.fau.edu/index.php?main=1&nav=635

Kagen, P. N., Smith, M. C., Cowling, R., & Chinn, P. (2009). A nursing manifesto: An emancipatory call for nursing knowledge development, conscience, and practice. *Nursing Philosophy, 11*, 67–84.

Munhall, P. (1993). Unknowing: Toward another pattern of knowing. *Nursing Outlook, 41*, 125–128.

White, J. (1995). Patterns of knowing: Review, critique, and update. *Advances in Nursing Science, 17*(4), 73–86.

LEARNING RESOURCES

Dettmore, D., Kolanowski, A., & Boustani, M. (2009). Aggression in persons with dementia: Use of nursing theory to guide clinical practice. *Geriatric Nursing, 30*(1), 8–17.

Hoe, J., & Thompson, R. (2010). Promoting positive approaches to dementia care in nursing. *Nursing Standard, 25*(4), 47–56.

Jenkins, C., & McKay, A. (2013). A collaborative approach to health promotion in early stage dementia. *Nursing Standard, 27*(36), 49–57.

Jossee, L. L., Palmer, D., & Lang, N. M. (2013). Caring for elderly patients with dementia: Nursing interventions. *Nursing Research & Review, 20*(3), 107–117.

Locsin, R. (1998). Music as expression of nursing: A co-created moment. *International Journal for Human Caring, 2*(3), 40–42.

Picard, C. (1994). The power of dance. In D. Gaut & A. Boykin (Eds.), *Caring as healing: Renewal through hope* (pp. 146–149). New York, NY: National League for Nursing Press.

Sung, H. C., Wen-Li, L., Chang, S. M., & Smith, G. (2014). Exploring nursing staff's attitudes and use of music for older people with dementia in long-term care facilities. *Journal of Clinical Nursing, 20*, 1776–1783.

Weatherhead, I., & Courtney, C. (2012). Assessing the signs of dementia. *Practice Nursing, 23*(3), 114–118.

Williams, K. N., Herman, R., Gajewski, B., & Wiilson, K. (2009). Elderspeak communication: Impact on dementia care. *American Journal of Alzheimer's Disease and Other Dementias, 24*(1), 11–20.

CHAPTER 17

Caring Between a Nurse and an Older Adult in Hospice Care

This chapter presents a nursing situation focused on caring for a woman with intractable pain in a hospice care facility. Using the theoretical perspective of nursing as caring (Boykin & Schoenhofer, 2001), which focuses on enhancing personhood for the nurse and one nursed, the nursing situation highlights the aesthetic response to a call for nursing to provide relief from pain and suffering.

Directions: As you prepare to intentionally enter the world of the other, reflect on the following question: What are the expressions of caring between nurse and the one nursed?

NURSING SITUATION

Written by Patricia Blanchette Kronk, MSN, ARNP, GNP-BC

A SENTIMENTAL JOURNEY

One of our hospice patients had been in the inpatient unit several times for symptom management. We had developed a warm nurse–patient relationship, and I would often visit with her on days when I was not scheduled as her primary nurse. Once I was asked to make a house call to help her husband understand and organize her medications, as well as evaluate her status and level of comfort. Elizabeth was always kind and gentle, asking only for comfort. Her husband, Jim, was usually quiet, pensive, and supportive of Elizabeth. He wanted her to be as comfortable as possible. He told me that he would do whatever Elizabeth asked, and wanted to not be nervous or anxious in her presence. He admitted to me that his hardest moments in caring for Elizabeth were when she was in pain. He found it extremely hard to remain present and unable to do anything to relieve her discomfort. Both Elizabeth and Jim would seek admission to the inpatient unit during times of crisis; Elizabeth because she was desperate to be in pain control and equally distraught at the level of distress Jim suffered, and Jim because he was "helpless to help the love of his life." Both Elizabeth and Jim needed nursing care.

During what turned out to be Elizabeth's final admission to the hospice unit, I was privileged to experience many memorable moments with Elizabeth and Jim. Because Jim spent most of every waking hour at her bedside, leaving only for "real personal" personal care moments, I made sure I included him in conversations with Elizabeth. Over several weeks, I learned about their life and their love story. They spoke of falling in love, dancing to favorite songs of the Big Band Era, family, important times in their marriage, and the joy they experienced during travels around the world. Occasionally they would speak of a special time and then stop in their story, sharing an eye-to-eye conversation that was solely between the two of them. It was a privilege to witness these conversations and understand that my presence, while very real, was not noticed by either Elizabeth or Jim.

As Elizabeth's physical condition declined, we were all focused on comfort and symptom management for her. Nursing staff, the medical director, Elizabeth, and Jim were each and all focused on ensuring her comfort. The hospice care center provided a quiet room, comfortable bed, soft lighting, lovely décor, and garden view. Medications and physical comfort measures were provided around the clock by warm, caring staff. Elizabeth, however, was unable to achieve pain control, and was unable to sleep.

I remember one Friday afternoon, in particular, when I discussed Elizabeth's inability to sleep and intractable pain with her physician, several other nurses, and her husband. We were all concerned about her and I, as well as the others, vowed to find a way to help her. Around-the-clock pain medication dosing, as well as "prn as needed" for breakthrough pain, seemed inadequate. Her husband suggested that she just would not let go and let herself sleep. He had given her permission to let go, yet she remained awake, stoic, and the decision maker.

When I arrived on the unit the following Monday morning, I learned that she dozed only a few minutes over the weekend and that her husband never left her bedside. She remained awake that entire day, eyes open, rarely speaking, but offering a tentative smile now and then. We provided every comfort measure we could think of, with her permission, yet nothing changed.

Toward the end of my 12-hour shift, I went to her bedside to say goodnight. She whispered that her pain was unbearable, that she was "oh, so tired," and asked me to please give her another dose of her medication. Her husband stepped to the other side of her bed, took her hand, and said he would be a diversion until I came back with the medicine.

Just a few minutes later I dimmed the room's lights and started a slow IV push. I glanced at Elizabeth, who was looking directly at Jim, sharing one of their silent heart-to-heart conversations. I softly started singing a song popularized in 1944 by Doris Day, "Sentimental Journey."

When the dose was given, and the song was sung, Elizabeth and Jim smiled at each other; Elizabeth breathed a little sigh, closed her eyes, and drifted off to sleep. I turned to leave and found the entire staff gathered at the doorway, quietly listening. Elizabeth's husband asked, "How did you know that was 'our song'?" Of course, I did not know.

In reflecting on this nursing situation, I have wondered why I decided to sing during the IV push, and why did I sing that particular song? For me the call for nursing was to take Elizabeth out of her current suffering and back to a happier time. I had never responded to a call for nursing like this before. It came from deep within me, from a place of knowing of caring in nursing and of music popular during the Big Band Era when this couple would have been young adults. I was humbled by the impact this had on Elizabeth, Jim, and the hospice staff. Elizabeth taught me to be courageous and creative in my practice of nursing.

What were the calls for nursing? Certainly caring, comfort, authentic presence, and alternating rhythms come instantly to mind. First, though, is the question: How could I know what I was hearing on so many different levels? Toward the end of her life Elizabeth spoke very few words, and her husband became even quieter, yet they both seemed to cry out for help. As the honest caring and care provided by all seemed inadequate, I was personally perplexed by the need to do more within the hospice end-of-life structure. Why did I worry? Why could I also not let go?

My practice of nursing changed as a direct result of this nursing situation. I learned to trust my instincts, as this was the first time I really listened with the third ear when I silently asked, "What is really going on?" and "What are they really saying?"

Now, years later, reflecting on this nursing situation, I understand my novice approach to caring in nursing and nursing from the world of other. I was able to place myself in their shoes and better understand their wants and needs. Nursing as caring (Boykin & Schoenhofer, 2001) is the philosophy and model of practice for me.

STUDY PROCESS

The Barry, Gordon & King Teaching/Learning Nursing Framework process is a broad guide to study and analyze nursing situations, focusing on the caring between the nurse and person nursed. The following analysis guides and inspires understanding of nursing from the theoretical perspective of Nursing as Caring (Boykin & Schoenhofer, 2001), which focuses on enhancing personhood for the nurse and the one nursed.

What Was the Caring Between the Nurse and the One Nursed?

The nurse identified the following caring concepts—comfort, authentic presence, and alternating rhythms—that guided caring for Elizabeth. What other expressions of caring are present in the nursing situation? What mattered most in the moment to Elizabeth?

Using the Ways of Knowing, How Can We Come to Understand the Call(s) for Nursing?

How does each of the ways of knowing—personal, empirical, ethical, sociopolitical, spiritual, emancipatory, unknowing, aesthetic—inform understanding of caring in this nursing situation (Carper, 1978; Kagen, Smith, Cowling, & Chinn, 2009; Munhall, 1993; White, 1995)?

The writer of the nursing situation offers the following descriptions of the ways of knowing that guided her practice. What ways of knowing inform your practice?

Personal knowing: This is evident because of my many years in nursing practice and nursing education, but the heart of my personal knowing in this situation, I believe, stems from the time I was a teenager, watching my mother leave this life, and wondering what else I could and should do for her. She asked me to sing "Tell Me Why."

Empirical knowing: This is apparent in nursing education, graduate studies, continuing education, and specialty nursing education. Policies and procedures are a part of nursing life and provide guidelines for safe practice. We know what to do and how to do it. The standard plan of care, however, did not meet her needs.

Ethical knowing: This is evident because of the balance of right versus wrong, enough versus not enough in achieving comfort within the death and dying structure of hospice. Understanding the practice structure of the environment, and balancing what was right for this patient, her husband, and myself, freed me to dim the lights, sing a song, and answer the moral call to do more.

Sociopolitical knowing: What knowledge do you need to understand hospice care? What are the local, state, and national laws and regulations that govern hospice care? What are the admission criteria for hospice? What are the paying sources for hospice care? What is the community understanding and acceptance of hospice care?

Spiritual knowing: What are Elizabeth's spiritual beliefs and practices?

Emancipatory knowing: What knowledge is needed for understanding advance directives? What advocacy actions are needed?

Unknowing: As you reflect on the nursing care of Elizabeth and her husband, what are you feeling? What was communicated nonverbally to the family? How can the nurse be open to understanding Elizabeth's experience? What mattered most in the moment to Elizabeth?

Aesthetic knowing: Aesthetic knowing is at the core of understanding what happened within this nursing situation, in that the "whole" of it was experienced, felt, appreciated, and respected. Everything came together in those few minutes of singing an "oldie goldie" while the lights were low, and as the medication was slowly infused. Elizabeth, Jim, the ambiance created by the soft lights, medication, and me softly singing a song from their past that brought forth heart-felt memories of long ago all brought calm to a hurting person and helped her achieve relaxation and peaceful, pain-free sleep.

What Are the Calls for Nursing?

The nurse heard a distinct verbal call for pain relief both from Elizabeth and Jim. What are some possible variations in calls? What calls for nursing do you hear?

What Are the Responses to the Calls for Nursing Present in the Situation?

The nurse described checking the order and medication record and preparing the morphine. In a moment of full understanding of multiple ways of knowing, she created a healing environment by dimming the lights, administering the morphine IV push slowly, and then singing softly, "*Gonna take a sentimental journey.*" What other nursing responses are possible?

What Was the Outcome of the Response(s) in Relation to the Call(s)?

The nurse used nursing as caring (Boykin & Schoenhofer, 2001), which focuses on enhancing personhood for the nurse and the one nursed.

For the person nursed, Elizabeth: Elizabeth seemed soothed by the song, shared a smile with Jim, and drifted off to sleep free from pain in that moment.

For her husband, Jim. He shared an intimate moment—the smile—with Elizabeth and felt relieved she was able to sleep and have a break from the pain.

For the nurse: The nurse says her practice was changed forever. She learned to listen with a third ear so she could discern what was really going on and what they were really asking. She learned to hear silent calls for nursing from Elizabeth and her husband for rest. The nurse learned to trust her instincts, as she authentically listened and silently asked: What is really going on and what are they really saying?

For the hospice staff. They were drawn to the room by the soft singing and witnessed an exquisite expression of caring.

For the nursing profession. This nursing situation is retold and offers untold opportunities for understanding anew the impact of caring for the nurse, the one nursed, for Jim, and for staff and colleagues.

For others: What is the value of being cared for? How did Elizabeth and Jim experience caring? What is the value of spending your last moments on earth in a nurse's presence having your song lovingly crooned? What is the value of end-of-life care?

How Did the Study of This Nursing Situation Enhance Your Knowledge of Nursing?

What did I learn about myself as I studied this situation? What did I learn about caring science? What new possibilities can be created from this nursing situation?

LEARNING ACTIVITIES

Journal: Reflect on and describe what happened between the nurse and one nursed.

BOX 17.1   Reflective Journal

What are your thoughts on caring expressed by the nurse in this situation?

Aesthetic re-presentation: How can this nursing situation be aesthetically re-presented?

BOX 17.2   Aesthetic Re-presentation

How would you aesthetically re-present this nursing situation?

REFERENCES

Boykin, A., & Schoenhofer, S. O. (2001). *Nursing as caring: A model for transforming practice.* New York, NY: Jones & Bartlett Publishers.

Carper, B. (1978). Fundamental patterns of knowing. *Advances in Nursing Science, 1*(1), 13–24.

Florida Atlantic University, Christine E. Lynn College of Nursing. (2012). *Philosophy.* Retrieved from http://nursing.fau.edu/index.php?main=1&nav=635

Kagen, P. N., Smith, M. C., Cowling, R., & Chinn, P. (2009). A nursing manifesto: An emancipatory call for nursing knowledge development, conscience, and practice. *Nursing Philosophy, 11,* 67–84.

Munhall, P. (1993). Unknowing: Toward another pattern of knowing. *Nursing Outlook, 41,* 125–128.

White, J. (1995). Patterns of knowing: Review, critique, and update. *Advances in Nursing Science, 17*(4), 73–86.

LEARNING RESOURCES

Albom, M. (2002). *Tuesdays with Morrie: An old man, a young man, and life's greatest lesson.* New York, NY: Doubleday Publisher.

American Nurses Association. (2010). *Registered nurses roles and responsibilities in providing expert care and counseling at the end of life: A position statement.* Silver Springs, MD: Author.

Davis, C. (2001). *I knew a woman: Four women patients and their female caregiver.* New York, NY: Ballantine Books.

Day, D. (1945). Singing "Sentimental Journey." Retrieved from http://www.youtube.com/watch?v=PUw125JMVFI and http://www.azlyrics.com/lyrics/franksinatra/sentimentaljourney.html

Gaines, E. (1993). *A lesson before dying.* New York, NY: Alfred A. Knopf Publisher.

The Hastings Center Organization. (2014). *End of life.* Washington, DC: Author. Retrieved from http://www.thehastingscenter.org/Issues/Default.aspx?v=244

Melvin, C. (2008). Hospice referral: What takes so long? *International Journal for Human Caring, 12*(3), 24–30.

National Hospice and Palliative Care Organization. (2014). *Resource guide.* Alexandria, VA: Author. Retrieved from http://www.nhpco.org/resources/end-life-care--resources

Tolstoy, L. (1886/1960). *The death of Ivan Illich* (Translated by Aylmer Maude). New York, NY: New American Library. Retrieved from http://www.ccel.org/ccel/tolstoy/ivan.html

CHAPTER 18

Caring Among a Nurse Practitioner and a Parenting Teen and Child

This chapter presents a nursing situation focused on the caring between a nurse practitioner, a parenting teen, and her baby in a school-based health clinic. Using the philosophical perspective of caring (FAU, CON, 2012), which focuses on nurturing the wholeness and well-being of persons in caring relationships, the nursing situation highlights the nurse's growing understanding of caring.

Directions: As you prepare to intentionally enter the world of the other, reflect on the following question: What are the expressions of caring between nurse and the one nursed?

NURSING SITUATION

Written by Mary Ellen Wright, PhD, APRN, CPNP

TALK TO THE HAND

Of all the clinical experiences that I've had in over 30 years of being a nurse, the "Camelot" of my career remains the opportunity to be the nurse practitioner and clinic manager of a school-based clinic for pregnant and parenting teenagers. Girls in middle school or high school who were pregnant could either stay in their current school or choose to attend a teen parent program during their pregnancy or after they became mothers. Included in the program were (a) bus transportation for the girls and their babies, (b) a day care for the babies, (c) an adult module-type education that prevented them from falling behind in class even when they had maternity leave, and (d) full health care services in the clinic that provided prenatal care, postpartum family planning, and pediatric primary care.

When I first started the clinic, I would go and meet the school buses every morning to meet the girls and their babies. It was an inspiration to witness the sea of girls, some pregnant and others struggling off the bus with a backpack, diaper bag, and a car seat with baby or a toddler holding on to their pant leg. I quickly realized after seeing the babies in the morning that the first few hours of the clinic needed to be focused on sick baby care.

One morning as I rounded in the day care, I observed a baby named James with respiratory distress, nasal flaring, retractions, and noisy breathing. I took James back to the clinic for a nebulizer treatment and called the school office to ask the mother to come to the clinic. When James's 15-year-old mother, Anna, arrived to the clinic, I was greeted by the palm of her hand in my face and her emphatic phrase, "Talk to the hand." I was in shock and didn't utter a word. That was a good thing because it gave me a few seconds to reflect before responding. In that few seconds, I thought how scared this young mother must be to want an immediate wall between us. Her head was turned the other direction so that all I could see was the creases of her palm and the back of her head. Once I was able to speak I said, "Okay, Anna, I don't know how to talk to a hand, but I would like to have the opportunity to sit with you and talk about James's breathing." Her hand dropped just a little as I continued, "James needs a treatment that will help him breathe better and it would help him if you cuddle him during the treatment." Her hand was down now and she had turned just a bit so I could see her profile. "This must be pretty scary for you to see James having a hard time breathing, so let's you and I see what we can do to help him." James was being held by the medical assistant, who handed him to Anna. Anna quietly followed me with James to an exam room and nodded agreement to start the nebulizer. I had her count his breaths with me before and after the treatment. I moved slowly and spoke with a reverence that added to the sense of calm after a storm. There were long silences that seemed natural and assisted in the promotion of a peaceful place. James responded well to the treatment; his respirations slowed and the signs of distress resolved. Anna was still not speaking. However, she watched James throughout the treatment and occasionally stroked his head as she held him in her arms. I reviewed the treatment procedure and had Anna demonstrate how to give the treatment. She did not utter a word.

We needed to watch James for the day to see if his respiratory difficulties returned and to continue the treatment plan, so I asked Anna if we could take him to the sick baby area for the day. I told her she could stay with James or go back to class. She decided to go back to class. I asked her to bring James back to the clinic about an hour before the end of school for a recheck. I rotated through the waiting room between patients, to see if she had arrived. I felt tense and nervous but remained hopeful that she would return with James voluntarily. I had to be patient to let her know that I trusted her and give her room to show caring for her baby. How much easier it would be to just take over the care of the baby, but this scared mother needed to have the opportunity to be trusted and not threatened. Finally, Anna came through the door holding James. He had no signs of respiratory distress. I had gone during my lunch and picked up a nebulizer machine for her from the American Lung Association, so James could have treatments at home overnight if needed. I showed her how to use the new nebulizer. She smiled when she saw James had his own machine and gave me a smile. She was able to repeat the signs of respiratory distress, count the baby's breaths, and understood the need to go to the hospital if the nebulizer did not help James's breathing. I asked her to come again first thing in the morning for a recheck.

Overnight, I could hardly sleep. I couldn't wait until morning to see them. I went to the buses and saw them disembarking. My heart jumped as Anna came right up to me and followed me to the clinic. James had no signs of respiratory distress and Anna proudly explained to me how she gave James a treatment last night and before getting on the bus that morning. I told her what a great job she had done. She smiled and gave the baby a hug. We continued to see James twice a day for the next week. Each day Anna talked a little more, and by the end of the week she began to tell me about herself. Her story included who she lived with, her multiple boyfriends, her jobs, and so much more. I listened without judgment and continued to tell her how great it was that she was coming to school and what a wonderful job she was doing with James. I told her when she was ready, I would like to offer her a health examination. After the second week, she made an appointment for her own examination. After her examination, a lab result indicated that she had a sexually acquired disease. When I tried to reach her I was told Anna was in jail. I called the juvenile detention center and spoke to the nurse practitioner at the clinic, who told me Anna refused treatment until she could talk to me. I told Anna that she needed to trust them to treat her. She agreed to treatment at the detention center. When I asked about James, she said her mother was caring for him and she taught her mother how to use the nebulizer. I asked permission to call her mother to check on James and she agreed. Within a week Anna came into the clinic with a house arrest ankle bracelet around her left leg. She came directly from the jail to see me and tell me all that happened.

Within a month Anna was bringing her friends to see me, telling them they needed to talk to me about their birth control needs and other health concerns. Over the next couple years, I continued to see Anna and James and her friends and family at the clinic. I had the great joy of watching Anna graduate with her high school diploma.

A few years later, I was in a retail store with my three children and saw Anna behind the register. She almost leaped over the counter to give me a hug. James was now in preschool. Anna was happy with her job, and had goals to continue her education and plans to move up in the organization in which she currently worked. As we were leaving, my children asked me who that lady was. I told them she was someone I had come to know. Nursing is the opportunity to come to know another through authentic presence, reflection, trust, and patience.

STUDY PROCESSES

The Barry, Gordon & King Teaching/Learning Nursing Framework process is a broad guide to study and analyze nursing situations, focusing on the caring between the nurse and one nursed. In caring for Anna, the nurse was open in coming to know her and focused on how she was living caring with her baby, James. The following analysis guides and inspires understanding of nursing from the philosophical perspective of caring (FAU, CON, 2012), focusing on nurturing the wholeness and well-being of persons through caring relationships.

What Was the Caring Between the Nurse and the One Nursed?

In this nursing situation, the nurse blended the following expressions of caring between Anna and herself: compassion, competence, confidence, conscience, commitment, and comportment. She stated the first encounter was scary for both of them as evidenced by Anna putting up her hand and hiding behind it and by the nurse's feeling threatened at first and then empathetic to the young woman's fear. Competence was displayed by knowing what the baby physically needed, in addition to the competence of interacting in a way that would not ignite what was already a tense situation. She did not always feel confident in this situation. She worried that Anna would not return and that James would not receive the needed care. The nurse had doubts about her ability to trust Anna and her ability to gain Anna's trust. She also didn't always have trust in how she was performing as nurse, which led to a sense of insecurity. Trust is difficult to achieve when so much is at stake. Trust was eventually established through the growth of the relationship and coming to know each other. In the beginning of the relationship, every word and every action seemed magnified with a heightened conscience. The relationship was so fragile that it felt like any wrong move or word would shatter the possibility of coming to know Anna. Both Anna and the nurse displayed commitment to developing this relationship. The nurse continued to be open to her and she continued to reach out to the nurse and was open to her care. She demonstrated caring for the nurse by continuing to return to see her and bringing others to the clinic. Comportment was present by keeping a calm, professional atmosphere, despite the initial personal reaction of Anna's request to "talk to the hand."

The essence of caring in this nursing situation is trust. Being present, patient, and reflective provided the opportunity to come to know the other person and build trust. The nurse feels so privileged to have had the opportunity for she and Anna to come to know each other.

Using the Ways of Knowing, How Can We Come to Understand the Call(s) for Nursing?

How do the ways of knowing—personal, empirical, ethical, sociopolitical, spiritual, emancipatory, unknowing, aesthetic—inform your understanding of caring in this nursing situation (Carper, 1978; Kagen, Smith, Cowling, & Chinn, 2009; Munhall, 1993; White, 1995)?

Personal knowing: How did I live caring? How can I know Anna as a caring person? How will this experience deepen my understanding of finding courage to reach out to other parenting teens?

Empirical knowing: What knowledge is needed to care for a parenting teen or baby experiencing respiratory distress? What complementary modalities might be helpful for Anna or James? What therapeutic communication techniques would be beneficial to enhancing the wholeness and well-being? What knowledge from other disciplines could enhance one's understanding of persons caring for a baby with respiratory distress while managing the stressors of being a teen parent? What knowledge of school nursing is needed to care for parenting teens at a school-based health center?

Ethical knowing: Did the theoretical lens guide the nurse's ethical practice? What ethical principles are present in this nursing situation? How do codes of ethics guide nursing practice?

Spiritual knowing: How could the nurse support Anna's spiritual beliefs and practices?

Sociopolitical knowing: What is the context of Anna's life—school, friends, work, recreational activities, community monitoring? How do Anna's cultural beliefs impact her health and well-being? Who are her family members? Do they live nearby or at a distance? How does Anna's family support her as she goes to school and cares for James? How is teen parenting viewed within her family structure, culture, and society? What legal issues are present in this situation? What are the rules and regulations that govern school-based health clinics?

Unknowing: How could the nurse remain open to understanding Anna's hopes and dreams? What matters most to Anna at this moment?

Emancipatory knowing: Are there policies in place that affect Anna's wholeness and well-being? Does the nurse need to advocate for Anna to continue to attend school while caring for James? What policies direct the care of babies experiencing respiratory distress while the mother is attending classes or riding the school bus?

Aesthetic knowing: What is the beauty of nursing in this nursing situation? How could this nursing situation be re-presented aesthetically?

What Are the Calls for Nursing?

The nurse states that she recognized Anna's "talk to the hand" behavior as a fear response to James's respiratory distress and Anna's concerns about providing the care her baby needed. The nurse understood that overcoming fear and being trusted to care for James mattered most to Anna at that time. What other calls may be present?

What Are the Responses to the Calls for Nursing Present in the Situation?

The nurse responded to the call for nursing with courage, competence, comportment, compassion, authentic presence, patience, reflection, and a commitment to build trust. What other nursing responses could be created?

What Was the Outcome of the Response(s) in Relation to the Call(s)?

The nurse used the philosophical perspective of caring (FAU, CON, 2012), which focuses on nurturing the wholeness and well-being of persons in caring relationships.

For the person nursed, Anna: What mattered most for Anna was overcoming fear and being trusted to care for James. She was transformed by building a trusting, caring relationship with the nurse who supported Anna's ability to care for James, her family and friends, and herself.

For the advanced nurse practitioner: The nurse was transformed by coming to know Anna, trusting in her own ability to care for Anna and James, and guiding advanced practice focused on attending to what matters most for the person nursed.

For the nursing profession: The professional practice of advanced nursing is transformed by the exquisite example of intentionality to care in which the nurse sees through a veil of fear to appreciate caring in others.

For others: What is the value of being cared for? Caring for parenting teens in school-based centers supports their ability to care for self and their children.

How Did the Study of This Nursing Situation Enhance Your Knowledge of Nursing?

What did I learn about myself as I studied this situation? What did I learn about caring science? What new possibilities can be created from this nursing situation?

LEARNING ACTIVITIES

Journal: Reflect on this nursing situation and how trust, compassion, competence, confidence, conscience, commitment, and comportment nurtured wholeness and well-being for Anna and James.

BOX 18.1   Reflective Journal

Reflect on this nursing situation and how trust, compassion, competence, confidence, conscience, commitment, and comportment nurtured wholeness and well-being for Anna and James.

Aesthetic re-presentation: How can this nursing situation be aesthetically re-presented?

BOX 18.2   Aesthetic Re-presentation

How would you aesthetically re-present this nursing situation?

Movie review: View the movie *Precious* (Daniels, 2009). How does the lead character's experience inform your understanding of teen parenting?

BOX 18.3   Movie Review

View the movie *Precious* (Daniels, 2009). How does the lead character's experience inform your understanding of teen parenting?

REFERENCES

Carper, B. (1978). Fundamental patterns of knowing. *Advances in Nursing Science, 1*(1), 13–24.

Daniels, L. (Producer), & Daniels, L. (Director). (2009). *Precious* [Motion Picture]. Santa Monica, CA: Lionsgate.

Florida Atlantic University, Christine E. Lynn College of Nursing. (2012). *Philosophy.* Retrieved from http://nursing.fau.edu/index.php?main=1&nav=635

Kagen, P. N., Smith, M. C., Cowling, R., & Chinn, P. (2009). A nursing manifesto: An emancipatory call for nursing knowledge development, conscience, and practice. *Nursing Philosophy, 11,* 67–84.

Munhall, P. (1993). Unknowing: Toward another pattern of knowing. *Nursing Outlook, 41,* 125–128.

White, J. (1995). Patterns of knowing: Review, critique, and update. *Advances in Nursing Science, 17*(4), 73–86.

LEARNING RESOURCES

Asheer, S., Berger, A., Meckstroht, A., & Kisker Keating, B. (2014). Engaging pregnant and parenting teens: Early challenges and lessons learned from the evaluation of adolescent pregnancy prevention approaches. *Journal of Adolescent Health, 54*(3), 84–91.

Barry, C. D., & Gordon, S. C. (2005). Caring for students in school using a community nursing practice model. *International Journal for Human Caring, 9*(3), 38–42.

Broussard, A., & Broussard, B. (2009). Designing and implementing a parenting resource center for pregnant teens. *The Journal of Perinatal Education, 18*(2), 40–47. doi:10.1624/105812409X426323

Kirse, D. J. (2006). Infant with noisy breathing. *AAO-HNSF Patient of the Month Program, 36*(2), 1–28.

Schaffer, M. A., & Mbibi, N. (2014). Public health nurse mentorship of pregnant and parenting adolescents. *Public Health Nursing, 31*(5), 428–437. doi:10.1111/phn.12109

Skinner, M. L., Mackenzie, E. P., Haggerty, K. P., & Robertson, K. C. (2011). Observed parenting behavior with teens: Measurement invariance and predictive validity across race. *Cultural Diversity & Ethnic Minority Psychology, 17*(3), 252–260.

CHAPTER 19

Caring Between a Community Health Nurse and a Young Family

This chapter presents a nursing situation focused on the caring between a community health nurse, a young woman, the woman's child, and the woman's husband. Using Leininger's Theoretical Perspective of Cultural Care Diversity and Universality (Leininger & McFarland, 2010), which focuses on cultural care congruence, the nursing situation highlights the authentic response to a call for nursing to be with and do with.

Directions: As you prepare to intentionally enter the world of the other, reflect on the following question: What are the expressions of caring between nurse and the one nursed?

NURSING SITUATION

WRITTEN BY BERNADETTE LANGE, PhD, RN, AHN-BC

CLARISSA'S STORY

Women in recovery are representative of a unique culture in their expressions of care beliefs, values, and lifeways. As a community nurse I have frequent nursing encounters with women who have substance use disorders (SUD). Through a community outreach program to decrease black infant mortality, I became acquainted with a woman who was 7 months pregnant. Clarissa had a long history of substance abuse and complex health issues. She claimed she was not smoking crack while pregnant but continued to smoke more than two packs of cigarettes a day.

According to Clarissa, she had been approached by several health agencies during the previous months to enroll her in a drug treatment program. She was adamant that her substance abuse was under control and she was following up with her obstetrician as advised. She was concerned about her cardiac history. She complained that her hands and feet were always cold and her doctor gave her pills for circulation. She felt her cigarette smoking was a better choice than crack cocaine. I told her I admired her strength to make such a decision but a treatment program could help her through the pregnancy and any withdrawal symptoms. I informed her that I had an ethical and legal obligation to protect her baby. I also had a moral obligation to honor her as a mother. She said she could see my point but wasn't ready to enter into a residential program and she was not using [drugs].

My initial assessment of Clarissa's needs was facilitated by her extensive knowledge about her medical history. She was able to converse as though we were colleagues in a cardiac unit. She said most of her health care experiences were negative because she was labeled as being a druggie. I did not judge her as a woman stigmatized by SUD. Although I had considerable experience of how the community could provide care for women with SUD, I told Clarissa that I felt she had a lot to teach me. She said no one had ever told her that and was surprised I was so honest with her.

Clarissa invited me to stop by whenever I was in her neighborhood. We had a coffee in her small, but very organized, and homey apartment. Her husband was several years older than she and was thrilled at the prospect of becoming a father for the first time at age 60-something. The first time I was introduced to him by Clarissa, he seemed suspect of my visit and asked her, in Spanish, if something was wrong. Clarissa assured him that I was there just to have a coffee. He began to work in the garden. Clarissa and I chatted for a bit more. As I was preparing to leave, I went over to him and said, "Thank you for your hospitality. Please let me know how I can help you and your wife prepare for your baby." I spoke in Spanish. He barely smiled and pointed to a wheelbarrow full of vegetables. He prepared a carton of vegetables and put them in the trunk of my car. As a community nurse with an understanding of the concepts of transcultural nursing, I accepted the gesture, described by nurse theorist Madeleine Leininger, as being the transition from stranger to friend (Leininger & McFarland, 2010).

Clarissa wanted to exchange cell phone numbers. She would call me frequently and we would discuss her reluctance to enter treatment for SUD as she would define herself as being clean. She was confident that she would continue to test clean in her urine specimens during her prenatal care. One day a dramatic change occurred as she developed false labor pains and went to the hospital. She called me and asked me to please come to see her as soon as possible. I met her husband in the hallway and he said, "They are saying that when the baby is born, they will take him away from her." He was very distraught and told me, "My sister will take care of my son but I don't want him taken away."

I visited with Clarissa and she was confident that her sister-in-law would assume parental responsibility if necessary. She was concerned about waiting in the hospital to go into labor and was anxious to go home. The cardiologist and obstetrician wanted her to be transferred to a high risk obstetrics unit in another hospital. Her obstetrician implored me to convince her to be patient while transfer arrangements were made. I told Clarissa that if she voluntarily entered a treatment program we could arrange for the delivery and she could enter a program with her baby. I also explained to her that part of treatment would be to learn parenting skills that would help her to retain parental rights. She told me she respected my opinion but it wasn't the right choice for her. She agreed to be transferred to a high risk maternal unit in the morning.

The following morning, I was informed that Clarissa had signed out AMA (against medical advice) in the middle of the night. I was unable to reach her by phone, she was not at home, and I could not find her on the streets she usually frequented. Later in the day I received a call from her. She said she was too uptight to stay in the hospital for fear she would go into labor and her baby would be taken from her. She also wanted to be able to smoke cigarettes. She told me she was just too edgy to not be able to smoke and had to leave. I respected her decision although I told her I did not agree. She said that was what she liked best about me, "You just tell me like it is."

During the next few days, we spoke on the phone regularly. She was working with a social worker to help prepare the papers for her sister-in-law to assume the parental rights. Clarissa and her husband were satisfied with the arrangement. Clarissa went into labor and had an uncomplicated delivery of a healthy baby boy at the local hospital.

More than 2 years have passed and I occasionally see Clarissa walking on the street. One day she invited me for a coffee to her new home. She and her husband have been displaced due to the hurricanes and now live in a motel. Locally, the motel has a reputation of being a "powder motel," where crack cocaine is sold. Clarissa has done wonders with their room. A small kitchen area is full of aromas of home cooking. She is anxious to show me a recent photo of her son. He is thriving in the care of her sister-in-law. I tell her that her enrollment in a treatment program could help her regain parental rights of her son. She assures me she is in control of how much crack she is smoking. She reminds me that I have not changed as I continue to tell her like it is.

STUDY PROCESSES

The Barry, Gordon & King Teaching/Learning Nursing Framework process is a broad guide to study and analyze nursing situations, focusing on the caring between the nurse and one nursed. Caring concepts that bring nursing to life and the multiple ways of knowing needed to care for this woman are the central focus of this nursing situation. Caring within Leininger's Theoretical Perspective of Cultural Care Diversity and Universality (2010) provides the inspiration for a new and different understanding of individuals.

What Was the Caring Between the Nurse and the One Nursed?

The nurse's caring for Clarissa is understated and yet illuminated with the thoughtful, respectful description of Clarissa as a person, woman, mother-to-be, mother, homemaker, and wife. She always referred to her by name and encouraged the steps Clarissa was taking for her baby's and her own health. Using alternating rhythms, the nurse stepped in close and stepped back reflecting the ebb and flow of their relationship. What are the possible expressions of caring? What expressions of caring did you identify as you read the nursing situation?

Using the Ways of Knowing, How Can We Come to Understand the Call(s) for Nursing?

How does each of the ways of knowing—personal, empirical, ethical, sociopolitical, spiritual, emancipatory, unknowing, aesthetic—inform understanding of caring in this nursing situation (Carper, 1978; Kagen, Smith, Cowling, & Chinn, 2009; Munhall, 1993; White, 1995)?

Personal knowing: The nurse's understanding of self as caring person supported her understanding of other's expressions of caring. How does the nurse's understanding of self influence her understanding of Clarissa as a caring person? How can she be helpful to Clarissa and her family? How can she be helpful to others?

Empirical knowing: What does the nurse need to know about women in recovery? What research has been conducted on this topic that can contribute to understanding? How can the caring concepts of courage and compassion guide the nurse? How does Leininger's theoretical lens promote a broad understanding of the culture of women in recovery? What does the nurse need to know about upstream thinking to facilitate community caring?

Ethical knowing: The nurse's care was grounded in ethical knowing by urging Clarissa to seek help and yet remaining true to supporting Clarissa's choices. How do codes for nurses provide a foundation for ethical practice? How should women in recovery be supported and cared for?

Sociopolitical knowing: What are the social determinants of health? How do they impact our understanding of caring for vulnerable and marginalized groups? What are the local, state, and federal policies and laws that impact recovery for women?

Spiritual knowing: What are the faith-based resources in the community for women?

Emancipatory knowing: What is the role of nursing in advocating for the rights of women in recovery?

Unknowing: How can the nurse build a trusting relationship with a woman in recovery? How can the nurse uncover what matters most for the woman?

Aesthetically knowing: How can the beauty of this nursing situation be re-presented in an art form? What other sources of knowledge would be helpful for the nurse in caring for Clarissa?

What Are the Calls for Nursing?

The nurse heard a distinct call from Clarissa to support her choices about wholeness and well-being for herself and her baby. What calls for nursing do you hear?

What Are the Responses to the Calls for Nursing Present in the Situation?

The nurse shared her deep knowing of community health, culturally congruent care, community resources, and how to be respectfully real. She was concerned for Clarissa and responded to her calls for nursing by being present each time Clarissa invited the nurse to be with her, whether it be in her home, her hospital room, or on the street. The nurse felt connected to Clarissa and Clarissa voiced the same connection to the nurse. Leininger asserts there are several concepts that are universally acknowledged by many individuals of diverse cultural groups. They are respect, concern, being there, feeling a connection, protecting, touching, helping, assisting, and facilitating. What are some possible variations in creating a response? How would you have responded?

What Was the Outcome of the Response(s) in Relation to the Call(s)?

The nurse states she was guided by Culture Care Diversity and Universality (Leininger & McFarland, 2010). How do the outcomes reflect the purpose of the theoretical lens? In what way were the nurse's actions culturally competent? How did the care reflect the three care modes: culture care preservation, culture care accommodation, or culture care repatterning that is beneficial, satisfying, and meaningful to Clarissa and her family (Leininger & McFarland, 2010, p. 334)?

For the one nursed, Clarissa: Clarissa seemed uplifted by the nurse's admiration for her choice to stop using. And she said health care workers usually just call her a junkie.

For Clarissa's husband: He was worried about the nurse's visits but learned that she was there to help and support. He showed his appreciation by placing a bushel of vegetables in the nurse's trunk.

For the nurse: The nurse says her practice was changed when she accepted the vegetables. She describes this gesture of gratitude as being the transition from stranger to friend.

For the community workers: They knew Clarissa was under the watchful eye of the nurse. They also knew the nurse and Clarissa shared a respectful appreciation of each other—each telling the other just how it was for each of them.

For the nursing profession: This nursing situation is retold and offers untold opportunities for understanding anew the impact of caring in the community from the theoretical lens of culture care that is meaningful and beneficial for the nurse, the one nursed, for the family, and colleagues.

For others: What is the value of being cared for? What is the impact of caring and supporting women in recovery on economics, safety, health, education, and the overall well-being of the community?

How Did the Study of This Nursing Situation Enhance Your Knowledge of Nursing?

What did I learn about myself as I studied this situation? What did I learn about caring science? What new possibilities can be created from this nursing situation?

LEARNING ACTIVITIES

Journal: Reflect on what happened between the nurse and the one nursed, focusing on nurturing and supporting persons in recovery.

BOX 19.1   Reflective Journal

Write your reflection on what happened between the nurse and the one nursed, focusing on nurturing and supporting persons in recovery.

Aesthetic re-presentation: How can this nursing situation be aesthetically re-presented? What image might depict this nursing situation?

BOX 19.2   Aesthetic Re-presentation

How would you aesthetically re-present this nursing situation?

REFERENCES

Carper, B. (1978). Fundamental patterns of knowing. *Advances in Nursing Science, 1*(1), 13–24.

Florida Atlantic University, Christine E. Lynn College of Nursing. (2012). *Philosophy*. Retrieved from http://nursing.fau.edu/index.php?main=1&nav=635

Kagen, P. N., Smith, M. C., Cowling, R., & Chinn, P. (2009). A nursing manifesto: An emancipatory call for nursing knowledge development, conscience, and practice. *Nursing Philosophy, 11*, 67–84.

Leininger, M. M., & McFarland, M. R. (2010). The theory of cultural care diversity and universality. In M. Parker & M. Smith (Eds.), *Nursing theories & nursing practice* (3rd ed., pp. 317–336). Philadelphia, PA: F.A. Davis.

Munhall, P. (1993). Unknowing: Toward another pattern of knowing. *Nursing Outlook, 41*, 125–128.

White, J. (1995). Patterns of knowing: Review, critique, and update. *Advances in Nursing Science, 17*(4), 73–86.

LEARNING RESOURCES

Barry, C. D., Gordon, S. C., & Lange, B. (2007). The usefulness of the Community Nursing Model in school based community wellness centers: Voices from the U.S. and Africa. *Research and Theory for Nursing Practice: An International Journal, 21*(3), 174–184.

Barry, C. D., Lange, B., & King, B. (2011). Women alive: Gathering underserved women upstream for a comprehensive breast health program. *Southern Online Journal of Nursing Research, 11*(1), 1–11. Retrieved from http://www.resourcenter.net/images/snrs/files/sojnr_articles2/Vol11Num01Art07.html

Butterfield, P. G. (1990). Thinking upstream: Nurturing a conceptual understanding of the societal context of health behavior. *Advances in Nursing Science, 12*(2), 1–8.

Lange, B. (2006). Mutual moral caring actions: A framework for community nursing practice. *Advances in Nursing Science, Philosophy and Ethics, 29*(2), E44–E55.

Lange, B. (2007a). A creative approach to disseminating research findings about women in recovery. *Substance Abuse, 28*(1), 51.

Lange, B. (2007b). The prescriptive power of caring for self: Women in recovery from substance use disorders. *International Journal of Human Caring. 11*(2), 74–80.

Lange, B. (2011). Co creating a communicative space to develop a mindfulness meditation manual for women in recovery from substance abuse. *Advances in Nursing Science, 34*(3), E1–E13.

Lange, B., & Greif, S. (2011). An emic view of caring for self: Grandmothers who care for children of mothers with substance use disorders. *Special Edition Advances in Community and Family Health, Contemporary Nurse: Health Care Across the Life Span, 40*(1), 15–26.

Zerwekh, J. V. (2000). Caring on the ragged edge: Nursing persons who are disenfranchised. *Advances in Nursing Science, 22*(4), 47–61.

CHAPTER 20

Caring During the Ebola Outbreak in Uganda

This chapter presents a nursing situation focused on caring for individuals suffering with Ebola during the outbreak in Uganda in 2000. This nursing situation highlights authentic presence despite struggling to be with and do for individuals suffering from an extremely virulent virus with a very high mortality rate. The following analysis guides and inspires understanding of nursing from the philosophical perspective of caring (FAU, CON, 2012), focusing on nurturing the wholeness and well-being of persons in caring relationships.

Directions: As you prepare to intentionally enter the world of the other, reflect on the following question: What are the expressions of caring between nurse and the one nursed?

NURSING SITUATION

Written by Fortunate Atwine, MNsc, RN, ICN

AUTHENTIC PRESENCE AMIDST A DEADLY OUTBREAK

My nursing situation takes us back to October 2000, when Mbarara Hospital experienced the first terrifying epidemic of the highly infectious disease of Ebola. Ebola is an extremely contagious acute disease that is usually fatal and is spread through contact with bodily fluids of infected persons. There are no known cures and the disease has a mortality rate of up to 90% (World

Health Organization, 2000, 2014). Based on this empirical body of knowledge at the time of the outbreak, there was a gap in the body of practical nursing knowledge. In Uganda, nursing is values-based and described as the main organizer of practical nursing knowledge. Practical nursing knowledge is characterized as the integration of values and core beliefs that are lived out in procedural actions. Nursing science is the main organizer of collective theoretical knowledge that guides practice (Uganda Nurses and Midwives Council, 2014).

The nursing and medical knowledge deficit of prevention and control of Ebola contributed to the widespread fear among health workers caring for and managing cases of individuals infected with the virus. The fear of becoming a contact person, an individual who is exposed to persons with Ebola but who has not yet exhibited signs and symptoms of the disease, was rampant. It was known that by the time a patient was diagnosed with Ebola, it was too late to provide ample protection against contraction of this deadly disease. When the diagnosis was made, a state of panic arose because protection had not been reinforced, and it was believed at that time that all the health workers who had direct contact with the patient would contract the disease.

After the sad news that many patients, including nurses, were dying, and that a senior doctor in the Gulu hospital had died, fear and panic increased among all nurses who were randomly chosen to work in the isolation unit. A care team of five nurses and doctors were assigned to provide all patient care in the isolation unit. The Centers for Disease Control (CDC) from the United States set up a resource site in Gula, ground zero for Ebola in Uganda, with laboratory services and health information. Personal protective gear was provided to health care workers in Mbarara, several hours away. We cared for five patients suffering with Ebola and sadly they all succumbed. The outbreak was contained in 3 months with the combined efforts of the nurses and doctors caring for the patients and themselves and with vigilance of the community health department's team in identification and surveillance of contacts. Seventeen nurses died of Ebola in Uganda but none from our hospital in Mbarara.

The poignancy of providing care while facing a life-threatening illness was palpable among the nurses. This contemporary event almost challenged the Code of Professional Practice from the Republic of Uganda (2008), and the International Council for Nurses Code of Ethics for Nurses (revised in 2012) that outlines the nursing profession's commitment to respect, promote, protect, and uphold the fundamental rights of people who are both the recipients and providers of nursing and health care. This nursing situation represents the lived experience for patients and the health workers in the Ebola isolation unit of finding balance between waiting to know and hoping for life, while at the same time anticipating death.

STUDY PROCESS

The Barry, Gordon & King Teaching/Learning Nursing Framework process is a broad guide to study and analyze nursing situations, focusing on the caring between the nurse and one nursed. Caring concepts that bring nursing to life and the multiple ways of knowing needed to care for this population are the central focus of this nursing situation. The theoretical perspective used to guide this nursing situation is King's Theory of Goal Attainment (King, Sieloff, Killeen, & Frey, 2010), which focuses on mutual goal setting between the nurse and the one nursed, contributing to wholeness and the attainment of goals of health or peaceful death.

What Was the Caring Between the Nurse and the One Nursed?

The nurse's expressions of caring were not focused on an individual but rather on the population of individuals infected with Ebola hospitalized at a regional hospital in Uganda. The gap of empirical medical and practical nursing knowledge was a challenge. However, the Code of Professional Practice from the Republic of Uganda (Uganda Nurses and Midwives Council, 2014) and the International Council for Nurses Code of Ethics for Nurses (revised in 2012) grounded the nurse in the commitment to respect, promote, protect, and uphold the fundamental rights of people who are both the recipients and providers of nursing and health care. Further, the Ugandan Code of Professional Practice specifically adds that persons will be treated with respect despite HIV status or any other situation of vulnerability. What expressions of caring did you identify as you read the nursing situation?

Using the Ways of Knowing, How Can We Come to Understand the Call(s) for Nursing?

How does each of the ways of knowing—personal, empirical, ethical, sociopolitical, spiritual, emancipatory, unknowing, aesthetic—inform your understanding of caring in this nursing situation (Carper, 1978; Kagen, Smith, Cowling, & Chinn, 2009; Munhall, 1993; White, 1995)?

In this nursing situation, the nurse shared her deep knowing of the Code for Nursing Ethics in Uganda and Australia and used these as her anchor to provide respectful care on the isolation unit of the regional hospital. King and colleagues (2010) assert that goals toward wholeness and health are mutually developed by the nurse and one nursed as each lived fearfully of the diagnosis and prognosis in this nursing situation.

Personal knowing: What do I need to know about myself and the one nursed or the potential population of persons infected with Ebola? Who am I as a caring person? How am I living caring as a professional nurse? How is the one nursed living caring? What personal knowledge do I bring to this situation? How does the virulence of this virus influence my caring in this unique situation?

Empirical knowing: What does the nurse need to know about Ebola, transmission, manifestation, incubation, and course? What does the nurse need to know about symptoms and treatment? What other sources of empirical knowledge would be helpful in caring for individuals infected with Ebola? How would a person's age, gender, and human growth and development level influence reactions to an Ebola infection? What does the nurse need to know about protecting self, colleagues, family, and community members? What are the *Millennium Health Development Goals* (World Health Organization, 2000)? What complementary modalities could be helpful in this situation: music, dim lights, guided imagery, relaxation, deep breathing exercises? What research studies have been conducted on the lived experience of Ebola?

Ethical knowing: How do ethical codes ground caring and keep health care workers focused on what is right and just? How do the values of the theoretical perspective guide nursing care in developing mutual goals and support wholeness for the persons nursed? Is the nurse honest and trustworthy? Is personal information kept confidential?

Sociopolitical knowing: What is the context of this person's life? Who are the family members? What cultural factors influence contagion, family care, and health-seeking decisions? What is the status of the ability to pay for services or health insurance coverage? How would a person feel about not being able to see or be cared for by family members? What are the issues surrounding identifying and isolating persons inflected with Ebola? What measures are needed to protect the public from exposure? What environmental factors may influence contagion? What local, state, and federal policies and laws are impacting care and containment of Ebola? What social structures impact the practice of nursing in this situation?

Spiritual knowing: What does the nurse need to know to support religious and/or spiritual beliefs and practices? What nursing interactions or transactions support or facilitate spiritual comfort?

Emancipatory knowing: How does an environment of patriarchy influence caring? Are there injustices evident? How can nurse advocacy influence goal attainment?

Unknowing: How can the nurse bracket what is known from the chart, reports, conversations, and news media to come to know others? How was the nurse open to understanding the nursing situation from the perspective of a person with Ebola? What are the person's goals for health or a peaceful death?

Aesthetic knowing: What metaphors or artistic expressions could represent nursing interactions and transactions? How can all the ways of knowing be woven into the fabric of understanding nursing in this situation?

What Are the Calls for Nursing?

The nurse heard a distinct call from individuals to provide care and support as they experienced the ravages of the Ebola virus. What calls for nursing do you hear?

What Are the Responses to the Calls for Nursing Present in the Situation?

The nurse responded with care and concern for the ones nursed as well as for herself and colleagues. She was on the same journey with the ones nursed, waiting to hear, waiting to know, and waiting for symptoms to emerge. What are some possible variations in creating a response? How would you have responded?

What Was the Outcome of the Response(s) in Relation to the Call(s)?

The nurse used the theoretical perspective of goal attainment (King et al., 2010), which focuses on mutual goal setting between the nurse and the one nursed, contributing to wholeness and the attainment of goals of health or peaceful death. In what way did the outcomes reflect this theoretical lens?

For the population of persons inflected with Ebola: The nurse stayed true to the code of ethics and provided care to the best of her ability. Treatment protocols were not available and caring interactions were developed on the spot in collaboration with the one nursed and the situation. Palliative interactions provided comfort to the ones nursed until death.

For the nurse: During the outbreak, the nurse carefully and conscientiously followed isolation protocols contributing to a safe environment for the health care team and all remained free of the virus. Following this outbreak, the nurse enrolled in a graduate nursing program to become more knowledgeable about expanding the autonomy and legal authority of the profession through education and research.

For the nursing profession: What can others learn about being a nurse and caring for persons infected with Ebola? What can be learned about living with compassion and finding courage in fearful situations? What is learned about caring for and appreciating nurse colleagues who are mutually setting goals with clients and journeying together toward health or a peaceful death?

For others: What is the value of being cared for? What can we learn about putting a human face on Ebola and understanding its impact on humanity? What is the impact of being cared for while suffering with unbearable symptoms of Ebola—living with hope but expecting the worst? How can physicians, social workers, and other health care professionals learn from this nursing situation and the commitment to uphold codes of ethical conduct?

How Did the Study of This Nursing Situation Enhance Your Knowledge of Nursing?

What did I learn about myself as I studied this situation? What did I learn about caring science? What new possibilities can be created from this nursing situation?

LEARNING ACTIVITIES

Journal: Reflect on and describe what happened between the nurse and one nursed.

BOX 20.1   Reflective Journal

What are your thoughts on caring expressed by the nurse in this situation?

Aesthetic re-presentation: How can this nursing situation be aesthetically re-presented?

BOX 20.2   Aesthetic Re-presentation

How would you aesthetically re-present this nursing situation?

REFERENCES

Carper, B. (1978). Fundamental patterns of knowing. *Advances in Nursing Science, 1*(1), 13–24.
Florida Atlantic University, Christine E. Lynn College of Nursing. (2012). *Philosophy.* Retrieved from http://nursing.fau.edu/index.php?main=1&nav=635

Kagen, P. N., Smith, M. C., Cowling, R., & Chinn, P. (2009). A nursing manifesto: An emancipatory call for nursing knowledge development, conscience, and practice. *Nursing Philosophy, 11,* 67–84.

International Council of Nurses. (2012). *The INC code of ethics for nurses.* Retrieved from http://www.icn.ch/images/stories/documents/about/icncode_english.pdf

King, I., Sieloff, C. L., Killeen, M. B., & Frey, M. A. (2010). Imogene King's theory of goal attainment. In M. Parker & M. Smith (Eds.), *Nursing theories & nursing practice* (3rd ed., pp. 146–166). Philadelphia, PA: F.A. Davis.

Munhall, P. (1993). Unknowing: Toward another pattern of knowing. *Nursing Outlook, 41,* 125–128.

Uganda Nurses and Midwives Council. (2014). Conduct/Ethics. Retrieved from http://unmc.ug/conductethics/

White, J. (1995). Patterns of knowing: Review, critique, and update. *Advances in Nursing Science, 17*(4), 73–86.

World Health Organization. (2000). *Millennium health development goals.* Retrieved from http://www.who.int/topics/millennium_development_goals/en/

World Health Organization. (2014). Fact sheet/Ebola. http://www.who.int/media centre/factsheets/fs103/en/

LEARNING RESOURCES

Centers for Disease Control and Prevention. (2014). *Information for healthcare workers.* Retrieved from http://www.cdc.gov/flu/professionals/

Harrowing, J. (2011). Compassion practice by Ugandan nurses who provide HIV care. *The Online Journal of Issues in Nursing, 16*(1), Manuscript 5.

Harrowing, J. N., & Mill, J. (2010). Moral distress among Ugandan nurses providing HIV care: A critical ethnography. *International Journal of Nursing Studies, 47*(6), 723–731.

Kyarimpa, J. (2009, April 6). Uganda: Village health teams—First draft of a solution. *Inter Press Service News Agency.* Retrieved from http://www.ipsnews.net/2009/04/uganda-village-health-teams-first-draft-of-a-solution/

Locsin, R. C. (2002). Ebola at Mbarara, Uganda: Aesthetic expressions of the lived worlds of people waiting to know. *Nursing Science Quarterly, 15*(2), 123–130.

Locsin, R. C., Barnard, A., Matua, G. A., & Bongomin, B. (2003). Surviving Ebola: Understanding experience through artistic expression. *International Council of Nurses, International Nursing Review, 50,* 156–166.

Locsin, R. C., & Matua, G. A. (2002). The lived experience of waiting-to-know: Ebola at Mbarara, Uganda. *Journal of Advanced Nursing, 37*(2), 173–181.

National Center for Emerging and Zoonotic Infectious Disease. (2015). *CDC Ebola fact sheet 2014.* Retrieved from http://www.cdc.gov/vhf/ebola/pdf/ebola-factsheet.pdf

Epilogue

Savina O. Schoenhofer

You, the reader, may be asking yourself, "Where do I start? Where do I go from here?" In reading the first section of the book, we have gained a beginning understanding of why we need to hear stories of nursing situations. The formalized literature on nurses' stories, stories of nursing situations, emerged with articles by Boykin and Schoenhofer (1991), Sandelowski (1991), and Benner (1991). Among influences on this literature were two books from disciplines other than nursing: *The Call to Stories* by Coles (1989) and *Narrative Knowing* by Polkinghorne (1988). Another influence on the value of nurses' stories was Carper's (1978) proposal of aesthetic knowing as one of the fundamental patterns of knowing in nursing.

The treasure trove of nurses' stories you have in your hands, *Nursing Case Studies in Caring: Across the Practice Spectrum*, is the first fully developed guide to using stories of nursing situations in teaching/learning nursing. In one of the chapters in this book, the nurse who contributed the story is said to have flipped the classroom, a growing approach to teaching in all disciplines and one that can take considerable courage, because it refocuses the orientation from teacher to student—with the teacher becoming a resource person and learners becoming the organizers of learning. For nursing faculty, experienced as well as novice, this reorientation can present a huge challenge. Most of us faculty teach in the same way we were taught, and may not be completely comfortable and successful in doing that. Using stories of nursing situations to teach nursing theory and practice does not require flipping the way you approach your teaching role. Stories of nursing situations can be integrated as part of the core structure of lesson planning, whether the method is cutting edge or traditional. So we ask again: How do we get started? And where do we go from here?

One aspect of this book that makes it so valuable is that chapters illustrate faculty using stories of nursing situations to facilitate teaching/learning in a broad range of nursing topics and pedagogical methods. There is no one way to most effectively arrange your teaching design to incorporate nursing situations. It is my good fortune to have used stories of nursing situations in the company of dedicated faculty colleagues, co-authors, and co-researchers for most of my teaching career. From this background, please permit me to offer a few suggestions on how to get started and where to go from here.

For me, the meaning of an instance of nursing *as* nursing is reserved and shared in a story that is guided by an explicit conception of nursing. For nursing faculty, the explicit conception of nursing that guides the curriculum of a nursing program—undergraduate or graduate—can be found in the curriculum documents, usually most broadly in the statement of philosophy and then elucidated in the curriculum framework, and made specific in individual course materials. Barry, Gordon, and King help us understand this idea in their early chapters that address broad nursing philosophical frameworks, commonly known as grand nursing theories. For nurse educators wanting to experiment with the use of nursing situations whose schools of nursing do not base their curriculum on an explicit grand nursing theoretical perspective, it will be important for you to study your curriculum documents carefully in order to generate a workable explicit conception of nursing to guide the structure of your nursing situations. In general, those conceptions will address in direct terms the nurse and one nursed, the form of relationship between nurse and one nursed, and the purpose for that relationship. Let me give you an example of what I mean.

The authors of this book are members of the faculty of a particular school of nursing. They have spelled out a definition of *nursing situation* that draws directly from the college of nursing's statement of philosophy: Nursing is the co-created lived experiences in which the caring between nurses and persons enhances well-being of persons and environment in caring. Additional curriculum documents further illuminate the philosophical and practical meaning of nursing and of nursing situations. My own practice in nursing education and nursing research is guided by an explicit grand theory of nursing, the Theory of Nursing as Caring (Boykin & Schoenhofer, 2001), and is spelled out as: "nursing is nurturing persons living caring and growing in caring," with a nursing situation understood to be a shared lived experience in which the caring between nurse and one nursed enhances personhood, with personhood understood to be living grounded in caring. These are just two examples of explicit conceptions of nursing that can be used to understand the meaning of a nursing situation. The key idea, for me, is that in order to work effectively with the concept of nursing situation, the concept of nursing has to be explicitly spelled out. I'll share just one more example that resonates with students in undergraduate and graduate programs of nursing; it is what I call the theory of nursing as medical assisting. I think you can see that any one of the three explicit models (Barry, Gordon and King; Boykin and Schoenhofer; and Medical Assisting) can be used to work with nursing situations, and that the focus and outcome of that work will be considerably different, depending on which of the three is used.

So, if you are wondering where to start and where to go from here, I encourage you to first clarify the conception of nursing you will be working from—whether it is a formalized statement from the curriculum documents, or from an explicit general theory of nursing, or even from a personal sense of nursing that has not been systematically analyzed and formalized (although I don't encourage the third path). Once you have a clear and explicit conception of nursing, then formulate a definition of nursing situation using that conception as a guide. In working with students using nursing situations, I have noticed that if there is not a deliberate working definition of nursing situation, the stories that are shared are often case studies or, at best, stories of nursing as medical assisting.

And where to go from the explicit conception of nursing rendered as a definition of a nursing situation? Use the definition to frame the writing of a nursing situation of your own experience and invite your students and colleagues to do the same. In sharing nursing situations, I have found it important to accept the stories with gratitude and to avoid a critique of the story as a proper story of a nursing situation.

In writing these stories, or asking others to write them, you can ask for specific circumstances—like location, age, medical focus, socioeconomic status, and such. However, the core of the story of the nursing situation would always be the same—a story of, in my case, shared lived experience in which the caring between nurse and one nursed enhances personhood.

I am grateful for the work of my colleagues, Barry, Gordon, and King, as a full treatment of the use of nursing situations for teaching/learning nursing. I look forward to the rich contributions you, the reader, make to the growing literature on this approach to teaching/learning nursing.

REFERENCES

Benner, P. (1991). The role of experience, narrative, and community in skilled ethical comportment. *Advances in Nursing Science, 14*(2), 1–21.

Boykin, A. & Schoenhofer, S. O. (1991). Story as link between nursing practice, ontology and epistemology. *Image—The Journal of Nursing Scholarship, 23*(4), 245–248.

Carper, B. (1978). Fundamental patterns of knowing. *Advances in Nursing Science, 1*(1), 13–24.

Coles, R. (1989). *The call of stories*. Boston, MA: Houghton Mifflin.

Polkinghorne, D. (1988). *Narrative knowing and the human sciences*. Albany, NY: State University of New York Press.

Sandelowski, M. (1991). Telling stories: Narrative approaches in qualitative research. *Image—The Journal of Nursing Scholarship, 23*(3), 161–166.

APPENDIX

Crosswalk Matrix

Chapter	Population	Physiologic System	Health Concern	Practice Setting	Caring Concept	Essential Concept
6	Older Adult Male and Wife	Cardiovascular System	CVA (stroke)	ER	Alternating Rhythms Authentic Presence Comfort Hope	Collaboration Communication Evidence-Based Practice Health Policy Interprofessional Professional Values
7	Young Female	Cardiovascular System: Hematology	Sickle Cell Crisis	ER	Authentic Presence Compassion Competency Commitment Empathy	Communication Evidence-Based Practice Health Care Disparities Organizational Policy Patient Safety Professional Values
8	Young Adult Female	Cardiovascular System	Cardiac Arrest/ Transplant	Acute Care	Compassion Competence	Evidence-Based Practice Patient Safety Professional Values
9	Adult Female	Gastrointestinal System Respiratory System	Cholecystitis Pneumonia/Ventilator	Acute Care/ ICU	Dignity Hope Love Patience Respect Trust	Advocacy Collaboration Evidence-Based Practice Health Economics Interprofessional Leadership Safety Professional Values Transcultural Care

10	Middle Age Adult Female	Reproductive System	Uterine Cancer	Acute Care	Authentic Presence Compassion Courage Listening Trust	Advocacy Communication Evidence-Based Practice Spirituality Professional Values
11	Newborn Baby and Parents	Death and Dying	Death of Newborn	Labor & Delivery/ NICU	Alternating Rhythms Authentic Presence Competence Compassion Courage Empathy	Collaboration Communication Evidence-Based Practice Patient Safety Professional Values
12	Child	Cardiovascular System: Hematology	Bone Marrow Transplant	Acute Care Oncology Unit	Forgiveness Love Patience	Advocacy Communication Professional Values
13	Older Adult	Neurological System	Transitional Care Chronic Mental Health	Psychiatric	Compassion Competence Courage Commitment Comportment Trust	Health Policy Leadership Professional Values
14	Young Adult Male	Cardiovascular System	Cardiovascular Disease Coronary Bypass Surgery	Transitional Care From Acute Care to Home Care	Authentic Presence Commitment Competence Listening Trust	Communication Economics of Care Health Policy Patient Safety Professional Values Leadership Transitional Care

(continued)

Chapter	Population	Physiologic System	Health Concern	Practice Setting	Caring Concept	Essential Concept
15	Adult Male	Urinary System	Chronic Kidney Disease	Transitional Care Kidney Dialysis Home Care	Compassion Competence Courage Commitment Trust	Advocacy Communication Evidence-Based Practice Health Policy Leadership Patient Safety Professional Values
16	Older Adult Male	Neurological System	Dementia	Long-Term Care	Commitment Compassion Trust	Communication Professional Values
17	Older Adult	Sensory System: Neurological	Intractable Pain	Hospice	Alternating Rhythms Authentic Presence Comfort	Advocacy Collaboration Health Policy Leadership Patient Safety Professional Values
18	Teenager	Respiratory System	Teenage Mom and Baby	Community/ School Nurse	Compassion Competence Courage Commitment Comportment Humility Patience Trust	Collaboration Communication Health Policy Leadership Patient Safety Professional Values

19	Young Adult Mom and Baby	Neurological System	Drug Addiction	Community	Alternating Rhythms Comportment Health Policies Humility Leadership Professional Values Trust	Advocacy Health Policy Leadership Professional Values
20	Community	Communicable Disease	Ebola	Acute Care	Compassion Competence Courage Commitment Comportment Patience Trust	Advocacy Communication Health Policy Leadership Patient Safety Professional Values

Index